Be the Rainbow

*

Bridge Heaven and Earth

How-to Manual for Integrating Alternative and Evidence-Based Medicine

by

Laura Kragie, M.D.

Laura Kragie, MD: Be the Rainbow • Bridge Heaven and Earth

Copyright © 2013 BioMedWorks® LLC

All rights reserved under International and Pan-American Copyright Conventions.

ISBN-10:14936007

ISBN-13: 978-1493600748

Laura Kragie, MD: Be the Rainbow • Bridge Heaven and Earth

PUBLISHER BioMedWorks® LLC

First Edition, April 2012

No part of this publication may be reproduced, distributed or transmitted in any form or by any means, or stored in a database or retrieval system, without the prior written permission of the publisher. Exception is made for brief quotations embodied in critical articles or reviews. Cover photograph is of the Vestmannaeyjar, Iceland volcano, © Fred Snijders, of Werkendam, Netherlands. Used with permission and appreciation. Cover design by Joleene Naylor.

DISCLAIMER: The information provided to the reader in this book does not represent a doctor patient relationship. Reader is advised to seek advice from their own personal physician. The information provided is only for informational and entertainment purposes.

As of publication date, the URLs displayed in this book link or refer to existing websites on the Internet. Publisher is not responsible for nor should be deemed to endorse or recommend any website (other than its own), nor any content available on the internet that is not created by publisher. The author, similarly, cannot be responsible for third party material.

This ebook is licensed for your personal reference and enjoyment only. This ebook may not be re-sold or given away to others (unless you have permission from BioMedWorks®) so please purchase an additional copy for each person with which you share it. If you are reading this book and did not purchase it or it was not purchased for your use only, then please return to purchase your own copy. Thank you for respecting the work and copyright of the author.

Laura Kragie, MD: Be the Rainbow • Bridge Heaven and Earth

DESCRIPTION

Just as the Rainbow connects Heaven and Earth, you can link Spiritual Practice and Mainstream Medicine. This book provides you with a cognitive scaffold that facilitates your mental ability to integrate Alternative Healing methods with those from Evidence-Based Medicine, thus allowing for the peaceful coexistence of the irrational with the rational. This manual is targeted mainly to physicians, to help them learn to work in teams that include Alternative Practitioners — and it's just in time for the start up of Accountable Care Organizations.

> *The intuitive mind is a sacred gift and the rational mind is a faithful servant. We have created a society that honors the servant and has forgotten the gift.* - Albert Einstein

Author and Rainbow Practitioner™

- Laura Kragie, M.D.

Dr. Kragie is a well-credentialed Physician and Scientist who has contributed significantly to both clinical practice and bench science. She was one of the first doctors in the United States to treat HIV/AIDS patients. Throughout her varied career in Translational Medicine she tested many different new therapeutics, using placebo-controlled clinical trials, to assess both their beneficial and harmful effects. She also compared new products to currently available therapies, including the alternative health practices.

See the website: http://www.biomedworks.com   for more information

Laura Kragie, MD: Be the Rainbow • Bridge Heaven and Earth

TABLE OF CONTENTS

PREFACE	i
BACKGROUND, PHILOSOPHY and INTENT	1
BRIDGE BUILDERS' TOOL BOX	3
BUILDING the SCAFFOLD	43
BASIC HOW-TO'S: RAINBOW PRACTITIONER™ LOGISTICS	52
THE TAKE AWAYS	64
NOW to LEARN MORE … SCIENTIFIC and CULTURAL TIDBITS	67
ACKNOWLEDGMENTS	113

Laura Kragie, MD: Be the Rainbow • Bridge Heaven and Earth

PREFACE

This book is a plain-speaking How-to Manual targeted to help primary healthcare providers, and less directly, their patients. It is not likely to be as pertinent to the trauma surgeon rescuing the accident victim or the emergency physician racing to head off meningitis in an acutely infected patient. But it will be of use to any and all folks who may be seeking a holistic approach to healthcare, and to better understand the characteristics of their health care providers.

Relief is sorely needed for many who suffer with chronic diseases that lack 'miracle cures,' such as — chronic pain, insomnia, headaches, arthritis, obesity, addictions, fatigue, weakness, dementia, affective disorders, attention disorders, high blood pressure, and angina — to name just a few. And U.S. healthcare costs are escalating. In response, the Congress enacted the Patient Protection and Affordable Care Act to change reimbursement policy, tying it to quality outcomes and cost efficiency. The Medical Homes practice model is but one newly created approach that emphasizes preventive and lifestyle interventions, and allows for the utilization of nontraditional, nonmedical staff. Another growing business model is the Concierge or VIP practice, which offers expanded time and resources to its clients. Ultimately, these practices seek holistic wellness, in order to reach better health quality, with decreased costs overall.

Patients and clients are spending billions of their own precious out-of-pocket dollars per year, on nonmainstream therapies. There is a pent up demand seeking relief that is not being met in the standard medical practice or hospital. Obviously, the healthcare establishment would be wise to address this 'alternate healthcare universe' and find ways to reconcile with it. If the two 'universes' could coexist, their combined practice would synergize healing for their shared patient, without increased expense. But how can logical, rational, doctors and scientists cooperate with these 'Heaven Helpers' who evoke magical forces, higher powers and fervent beliefs in the conduct of their healings? Science teaches skepticism and demands rigorous proofs, right?

This book offers you a cognitive scaffold to use to help tolerate that paradoxical mental duality of simultaneously using both science and belief, to heal. It outlines some basic fundamentals that are requisite for functioning as a Rainbow Practitioner™ — i.e., one who bridges heaven and earth. Most importantly, it proposes an Ethical Credo, essential for navigating the moral landscape inherent to practicing between and within the two worlds.

Please be clear, this is not a definitive scholarly treatise replete with extensive and exhaustive references. The ideas presented, however, are distilled from those of many scientists, philosophers, and inspirational figures from across the years and cultures. I leave it to the academic scholars to dissect out all the possible attributions. Instead, I direct you to this book's section titled, Scientific and Cultural Tidbits. There, you will find links to a mother lode of interesting, fascinating, comprehensible and entertaining material related to the general topics described in this Manual. I strongly urge you to follow your interests down these paths, and sate your curiosity. You will not be disappointed! In addition, please go to the website: http://www.betherainbow.com to find links to multimedia, podcasts, videos, slideshows, and notices for future workshops.

- Laura Kragie, M.D.

BACKGROUND, PHILOSOPHY and INTENT

Dear Readers, is it not our ultimate intent to relieve suffering, and enhance the healing of disease and injury in those fellow humans who seek our help? Here, I give you some mental tools to facilitate the path to this achievement.

If you plumb history, there are several brilliant visionaries who teach profound truths related to science, spirituality, ethics and religions. However, these thinkers are not easily available intellectually, to health practitioners and healers working in the trenches at the frontline of healthcare delivery. There is great need to synthesize these ideas, reduce them to practice, and create pathways to understanding for those of us involved in the daily struggle. The cognitive scaffold and toolsets presented here are pragmatic derivations of the teachings of Carl Jung, William James, and Albert Einstein, among many others. I combine their concepts, examples, and approaches into a more cohesive cognitive structure that will allow acceptance / tolerance / openness to healing-related irrational phenomena, in those who usually resist 'letting themselves go' into this area. I differentiate the traditional scientific toolset from those of these 'irrationals' and describe examples of where it is appropriate to use each and for which types of questions.

For simple clarity, I label the toolsets 'Earth' (for evidence-based medical practice) and 'Heaven' (for belief-based healing). The cognitive scaffold acts metaphorically as the 'Rainbow Bridge' connecting these paradoxical practices. It is derived from many sources. Myth, icons, metaphor, archetypes, imagery, music, anecdotes, and scientific 'tidbits' all attempt to illustrate a mindset / perception / perspective that has a capacity to embrace the irrational, experiential components, without compromising sound, rational intellect and judgment.

When we then combine 'Mainstream Medicine Doc' with 'Heaven Helper' we create the 'Rainbow Practitioner™'. This ethical healer is willing to navigate between and within the two worlds to best serve their client's needs. Utmost to the success of this 'Rainbow Practice' is an emphasis on the Ethical Credo: Duty to Distinguish and Disclose. The Rainbow Practitioner™ must be transparent at all times, and willing to distinguish the role and rationale they are assuming — 'Heaven' or 'Earth' — when dispensing therapy and advice. There should be no selling of snake oil and no pushing forth a pseudoscience.

Healers may span the spectrum from all-rational thought to the complete mystic. This book mainly teaches to physicians and scientists, but also speaks to alternative health practitioners and 'Heaven Helpers' from the healing professions. The cognitive scaffold and toolsets aim to facilitate the integration of faith-based beliefs with evidence-based medicine practice. Those two groups need to respect and utilize each other's different talents and skills, in the cooperative pursuit of wellness for their shared client. This collaboration will thus allow for a synergy of benefits to be made available to the client seeking relief.

> *The test of a first-rate intelligence is the ability to hold two opposing ideas in mind at the same time and still retain the ability to function.* - F. Scott Fitzgerald

BRIDGE BUILDERS' TOOL BOX

EARTH

'Earth' represents the evidence-based cognitive approach; ideally it addresses the when and how to appropriately apply the scientific toolset and to what kind of questions can best be answered with those tools. Star Trek's Science Officer Spock epitomizes the ideal stereotype for this type of thinking — fact driven, unemotional, detached, objective, rational, not intuitive and never 'gut instinct' driven. It is the opposite of 'Heaven' characterized by things like beauty, romance, emotion, mysticism, spirituality and ecstasy.

Evidence-based medicine uses the most current, available, best data to make decisions about the care of individual patients. It refers to clinically relevant research such as those examining the accuracy and precision of diagnostic tests, the power of prognostic biomarkers, and the efficacy and safety of therapeutic, rehabilitative, and preventive regimens. Randomized trials, and especially the systematic consolidated review of several randomized trials (meta-analyses), have become the gold standard to determine whether a treatment does more good than harm for a defined population. But evidence-based medicine is not just randomized trials and meta-analyses. For example, to find out about the accuracy and predictive value of a diagnostic test, we study an applicable cross-section of patients clinically suspected of harboring the relevant disorder, not a randomized trial. For a question about prognosis, we follow-up on patients identified at a uniform, early time point in the clinical course of their disease.

Sometimes the evidence we need, e.g. to better assess risk of toxicity, comes from the basic sciences like genetics or immunology. However, even excellent external evidence may be inapplicable to or inappropriate for an individual patient. Whether and where it should be applied depends upon how it matches the patient's clinical state, predicament and preferences.

THE EARTHY TOOLSET

SCIENTIFIC METHOD

The scientific method consists of systematic observation, measurement, experimentation, and the formulation, testing, and modification of hypotheses (theoretical, hypothetical explanations of the observations and measurements of the subject). It refers to a body of techniques we use for investigating phenomena, acquiring new knowledge, or correcting and integrating previous knowledge. With it, we gather empirical and measurable evidence that we can then subject to principles of logic. Deductive reasoning arrives at a specific conclusion based on generalizations. Inductive reasoning takes events and from them, makes generalizations.

Scientific researchers usually propose hypotheses to explain phenomena, and design experiments to test these hypotheses by studying the predictions (logical deductions from the hypothesis) that can be derived from them. Theories that encompass wider domains of inquiry may bind many independently derived hypotheses together in a coherent, supportive structure. Theories, in turn, may then help to generate new hypotheses to test.

Some essential elements of the scientific method include operations, observations, models, and a utility function used to evaluate the models. Operation is some kind of action performed on the system being investigated. Observation is what happens when the operation is done to the system. The proposed model is the fact, hypothesis, theory, or the phenomenon itself at a defined moment. Utility function is usually a measure of the model's ability to explain, predict, and control, the using of it. Any good scientific utility function is refutable and simple. The scientific method reasoning system is best used to discover phenomena which are subsequently understood in terms of new conceptual metaphors

— such as the metaphor of the "planetary orbit" model of the atomic nucleus and electrons, as was used by Niels Bohr.

For the testing of a drug in clinical trials, we define the null hypothesis to be tested as: assume two sample populations — treated versus untreated groups — are not different from each other and thus belong to the same original population. The null hypothesis is often the reverse of what the experimenter actually believes; it is put forward to allow the collected data to contradict it. We preset the statistics (significance tests) to define the boundaries where we can determine that the two sample populations actually originated from different parent populations (i.e. that the drug actually does have an effect), thus rejecting the null hypothesis, because the data did not support it. Usually that preset significance test is set at a 5% or 1% probability threshold that the results occurred by chance.

If the tests of significance determine that it is likely that the results do not fit the null hypothesis, then it is rejected, in favor of the alternative hypothesis. Otherwise, the null hypothesis is accepted. These are the only correct assumptions, and it is incorrect to reject, or accept, the alternative hypothesis. Accepting the null hypothesis does not mean that it is true. It is still a hypothesis, and must conform to the principle of falsifiability (its ability to be tested and falsified), in the same way that rejecting the null does not prove the alternative hypothesis.

Yet, many scientific discoveries were actually just stumbled upon, rather than deliberately sought out using scientific methods. Louis Pasteur said, "luck favors the prepared mind." Often the process of discovery starts with researchers finding bugs in their experiments. These unexpected results lead researchers to try and fix what they think is an error in their methodology. Eventually, the researcher decides the error is too persistent and systematic to be a coincidence. The theory, instead, was wrong, and new concepts to test are then born.

Laura Kragie, MD: Be the Rainbow • Bridge Heaven and Earth

RANDOMIZED CONTROLLED CLINICAL TRIALS

In medicine, we use scientific methods to design clinical trials, the predominant form being the Randomized Controlled Trial (RCT). The designs include:

- Parallel-groups: each participant is randomly assigned to a treatment group, and all groups are studied during the same time period. This controls for any events impacting the cohort during the time of sampling. Think of flu vaccination studies. Obviously the groups all must all have an equal chance of catching the seasonal virus in order to be comparable. Individually randomized, two-group, parallel trials are the most common type of RCT found in the medicine literature.

- Crossover studies: over time, each participant receives the experimental treatment, but follows a random order. This design reduces overall trial data variability because each subject serves as their own control, hence reducing the number of subjects needed to determine a significant difference between treatments. We commonly use this design for bioequivalence testing between drug formulations. But note, it would not work well for studies looking at factors that change significantly over time in the individual, like growth in children or the course of an infectious disease.

- Split-body studies: these look at different separate parts of the body of each individual participant (e.g. the left and right sides of the face) as randomized to receive a specific intervention. We commonly use these to study topical treatments such as pain ointments for arthritis or skin wrinkle treatments, where there is a symmetry to the disease manifestation.

The interventions to be tested in the RCT can be the experimental treatment as it is compared to a placebo control or to an active comparator treatment. The quality of the study data derived from the RCT is often dependent upon many factors. These include:

- Our ability to account for multiple influences simultaneously — isolating the impact of one factor while holding others constant.

- The extent to which the groups can be analyzed exactly as they existed when randomized into the trial. A "pure" intention-to-treat analysis is possible only when there is complete outcome data available for all the subjects randomized into the trial. When some outcome data are missing, e.g. from dropouts, we may be forced to only analyze cases where the outcome is known or else we use imputed data, like last observation carried forward (LOCF).

- Who was blinded after subjects were assigned to study treatments (for example, participants, care providers, those assessing outcomes) and how they were prevented from knowing the treatment and treated.

- Design and implementation of placebo control groups; whether there are sham treatments, double dummy, or untreated groups (which test the natural course of the disease or recovery of the cohort).

- The uncertainty associated with the data we collect; it depends upon the sampling method used and the frequency and number of samples taken.

But, even when performed optimally, there are still plenty of caveats to relying on the data from RCTs, including:

- Active comparator trials using the current standard of practice, can still be biased designs that disadvantage the competitor drug by using the wrong dosage, duration, or disease population; e.g. antibiotic trials.

- We cannot prove the negative or absence of an outcome, only can test to reject the null hypothesis using preset statistical parameters.

- Clinical trial extrapolation is limited; it tests a homogeneous population, with confounding subject medications and comorbid diseases excluded from the trial. The time frame is limited. Rarely ever is it equal to the real life situation for your individual patient. Way too much is still missing, and we cannot explain all factors and all scenarios.

- The sample sizes of many 'negative' RCTs are too small to make any definitive conclusions about the negative results — they are not 'powered enough' to conclude that there is no difference; instead is just a failed trial because it cannot make any conclusions.

- The clinical trials are very, very expensive and therefore they are not usually attempted unless there will be a major payoff to justify and compensate for their expense. That is why most trials only test new chemical entities that have solid patent protection and market exclusivity; generic compounds and those products that are already in the public domain are not examined, even if they are better therapies to use for the disease condition.

- Scientific Method and RCTs are very, very time consuming. And, they can be a gamble for the patients, with potential costs related to lost opportunities (i.e. patients could have chosen a standard active therapy instead of the chancy experimental one). It is an extremely inefficient method to use to make decisions. In reality, most minute-to-minute individual decisions are performed unconsciously and intuitively, and especially so with clinical decisions.

The perfect is the enemy of the good. - Voltaire La Bégueule (1772)

Dietary supplements, too, are 'drugs' but are not tested, not studied, and not subjected to quality assurance procedures, though they are still made on the same manufacturing equipment that stamps out the tablets for prescription drugs. Supplements may pick up traces of contamination from the shared manufacturing site ... and no one is checking those products.

Herbs and plant combinations are too complex to study using the earth tools such as RCTs. They consist of too many unknowable and changeable ingredients. The product is not consistent, not stable, and can have contaminants from the soil (like heavy metals) and the packaging. It is best to get your essential nutrients and ingredients from your daily meals. Rely upon your good, trusty, domestic, kitchen, farmer, and chef skills to evaluate your food and drink. (Hey, that's another earth toolset!)

Note, too, that we cannot use RCTs to test therapies used to treat fatal conditions. We cannot ethically use placebo controls in some situations such as cancer or lethal infection; instead we have to use cohort history or an active comparator to the experimental therapy, to test against. But the standard therapy used as a comparator may actually be ineffective; however if the new drug is shown to be 'noninferior' to that already approved standard, then it is usually approved for use, leading to just another ineffective therapy. We cannot use RCTs to test for rare events or for events occurring too many years out on the timeline.

Sometimes though, especially involving individual patients, an N = 1 is adequate. In an individual case, the hypothesis of a drug being responsible for an adverse event can be tested by repeating the suspected drug exposure in that same individual, but now controlling for all other pertinent variables (like other medications or suspect foods) and the experimental variable (the dose of the suspect drug) is varied systematically. Think of drug reintroduction studies to test for reappearance of an allergy or side effect, as an example.

RISK BENEFIT ANALYSES

An aphorism coming from the field of new drug development is, 'if you don't have an adverse event popping up along with your therapeutic effect, then you have not found it them yet ... keep looking.' We can crunch the numbers from study results and use them to figure out the number needed to treat (NNT) and number needed to harm (NNH). These help us to quantify how many patients we need to treat with one intervention versus another before encountering one additional patient who experiences a desired outcome (NNT) or an undesired disadvantage, such as a side-effect (NNH). (A smaller number indicates greater advantages for the NNT but greater disadvantages for the NNH.) Applying these simpler methods to complex research gives us a good indication as to whether, overall, a drug will benefit or harm our patients.

However, much of our clinical research literature comes from descriptive studies such as anecdotal case reports, case series, and cross-sectional surveys. Some come from a bit more analytical type reports like cohort and case-control studies which are observational — studies where the researcher reports whatever happens to be recorded as the outcome of treatment exposures. We can use the discipline of epidemiology to probe existing collections of observational and descriptive data, sussing out correlations that may generate hypotheses of possible associations of relevant factors to disease or adverse events. If variables are identified, sorted out and accounted for, then we may use case control studies to explore components contributing to relative risks. But do note that epidemiology studies such as these, give information on correlation and

NOT causation. We cannot assume items that group together are directly affecting each other, only that they seem to be riding along together in the same boat.

> *I consider that I understand an equation when I can predict the properties of its solutions, without actually solving it.* - Paul A. M. Dirac

Understanding the limitations of this powerful earth toolset is encouraged by the Ethical Credo: Duty to Distinguish and Disclose. We are obligated to acknowledge that clinical sciences alone may not be sufficient to solely dictate the best direction of our patient's care, and to disclose that knowledge when necessary. Here are a few examples of where earth tools can fall short:

- Statistics and quantitative information can be misinterpreted and manipulated (especially if there is profit to be made).

- Regression to the mean, thus reducing any apparent significant differences, can happen when you keep repeating the experiments and trials; we saw this happen with antidepressant clinical trials.

- Too many initial lab discoveries are not consistently repeatable, and do end up ultimately being a waste of time, effort and opportunity.

- There are some questions that cannot be answered with this earth toolset; e.g. interventions for otherwise fatal conditions, or situations that are too urgent to wait for the trials to be conducted, as in a public health emergency. And those questions that can be answered with it, are often too narrow and too restricted as testable hypotheses and verifiable applications.

- There can be a disconnect between the results of objective measures (e.g. FEV1) vs. subjective self-reported outcomes like symptoms, (e.g. asthma wheezing) where they do not correlate with each other. When this happens, it usually indicates a placebo effect is behind the improvements.

PLACEBO and NOCEBO EFFECTS

The natural course for many diseases, is that they seem to get better over time whether we treat them or not (e.g. depression). So we have to be sure to include in our studies, a test group where we provide NO treatment for comparison to those who are treated with the drug. Commonly, the folks we use for this group are those who pass through all the screening criteria, but are placed on the waiting list, and are not entered into the drug trial. Clinical trials also often use an initial placebo run-in preliminary phase to identify and sort out those subjects who do respond to the placebo, prior to starting the randomizing phase and initiating the experimental drug treatment; e.g. hypertension studies.

An illustrative example comes from reviewing the data of ~20 double-blind studies of clinical depression therapies — when the placebo group response was factored in, the larger contribution to therapeutic effect was actually attributed solely to the effect coming from placebo. Hmmm, what are the components of this potent and pervasive phenomenon, placebo?

Placebos can actually help cure people, or at least help them to feel better. Placebos — even when people knowingly take them — can work just as well as real drugs. And an effect of a placebo can persist for years. It seems that potent and powerful mojo comes along when using needle or knife. And the placebo phenomenon is shaped according to the personal symbolic universe of the individual patient. Somehow, the body is capable of reacting not only to direct physical and chemical stimulation, but also to symbolic stimuli, words and events that have special meaning for each individual.

We really do need to be aware of and understand this power of suggestion / belief in healing, because it does not always produce good effects. In fact, a nocebo is defined as a usually harmless substance taken by a patient that results in harmful effects when it is associated with the patient's negative expectations; it is the flip-side to the more desirable placebo effect.

Clinical trials testing pain relievers have taught us much about these placebo and nocebo effects. In patients who had been given a strong opioid painkiller, just "telling" them that their drug had worn off, even though the drug was still very much in their system, resulted in that person's pain returning to their pretreatment, predrug level. When the subjects felt that nocebo effect of pain, their brain scans actually showed them sensing pain.

The brain-imaging studies of clinical trial subjects showed that there is an expectation pathway involved with the placebo effect. Brain areas associated with sensing pain — the thalamus, insula and anterior cingulate cortex — lit up after a painful shock but was dimmed down in those patients who had been given the placebo treatment (that they expected would provide analgesia for them). Apparently their neocortex region increased in activity when patients expected that the placebo would reduce their pain. It seems their prefrontal cortex participated in their decision-making about how much pain they should expect to feel and how they should then respond to the painful challenge. If these patient's prefrontal cortex lit up in anticipation, thinking they would get pain relief, then their pain-processing regions of the brain cooled down; along with this, they actually reported feeling less pain.

So the placebo effect is truly different when it is compared to the effect of a typical specific pain treatment that acts by directly knocking out pain reception; instead it seems to be using a prefrontal top-down cortical influence upon the anterior cingulate cortex (limbic brain), similar to making an executive decision or judgment call. Those brain areas that do become active when we feel pain, such as the anterior insula and anterior cingulate cortex, these also activate when we know that someone we love is in pain. So these areas seem to be involved in the emotional and empathic aspects of our pain, as well.

Dopamine-related traits can predict a substantial portion of that placebo analgesia. Positive expectations lead to lower anxiety, and combined, these provide resilience — thus increasing the placebo, but decreasing the nocebo, responses. The orbitofrontal cortex is a brain region that is associated with processing evaluation and reward information, and it becomes involved in the emotional and motivational aspects of pain anticipation. Our desire for relief both amplifies expectations and strengthens placebo effects. It also conflicts with any expectations generated during nocebo interventions, and thus reducing those influences. These cognitive and emotional mechanisms mediate their influence on pain sensations via prefrontal-limbic-brainstem interactions.

Laura Kragie, MD: Be the Rainbow • Bridge Heaven and Earth

So, a patient's negative expectations do have the power to undermine the effectiveness of a treatment and to even produce the sensation of pain. But can nocebo kill? There is the famous case of ~100 Hmung young adult men dying of sudden death. These were Laotian refugees who had only been in the US for about a year. The Hmung community claims the culprit was a 'nocturnal spirit attack' but sleep paralysis phenomena, plus their cultural fear, plus genetics, are more likely.   Brugada syndrome, characterized by mutations and an abnormal EKG, seems to have caused the deaths; it is the major cause of Sudden Unexpected Death Syndrome and is the most common cause of sudden death in young Thai and Loatian men who are without any underlying cardiac disease.

And what about grief nocebo? Heart-attack survivors have attacks soon after the death of a family member or a close friend, more than at other times. This risk of having a heart attack declines as their grief slowly subsides.   Another real life nocebo zap is seen with Takotsubo cardiomyopathy, known as Broken Heart Syndrome because it occurs with intense stress and grief. These folks have cardiac myopathy and failure, but no obstructions in their coronary blood vessels to explain the cause, other than their profound sorrow.

UNWEAVING THE RAINBOW

Our loss of innocence from the Garden of Eden upon eating the apple from the Tree of Knowledge, provides a good analogy for when we gained our rational objective mind, but in the process, we lost touch with that paradise we had lived in, along with our wonder.

> *We have not the reverent feeling for the rainbow that a savage has, because we know how it is made. We have lost as much as we gained by prying into that matter.* - Mark Twain

Some apt metaphors depicting the inappropriate use of rational earth tools to examine questions from the irrational realm include Unweaving the Rainbow — both the God versus physics book (author Richard Dawkins) as well as Keat's famous poem. They lament the dismantling of essence and beauty in the pursuit of reductionistic knowledge. Reductionism ends up killing the entity under our study. A scalpel cuts the heart to pieces — it no longer beats, and ... no longer loves. Even Heisenberg's Uncertainty Principle states that when the event of interest is examined, it is changed by the act of observing it. And from Ken Pirsig's **Zen and the Art of Motorcycle Maintenance**, his main character, Phaedrus, futilely attempts to objectify, rationalize and define beauty, quality and excellence. He gets an answer to one question, but in the process creates hundreds more, much like the severed heads of the mythological Hydra, and they chase him into his own state of insanity.

> *When analytic thought, the knife, is applied to experience, something is always killed in the process.* - Robert M. Pirsig

The limitations of these earth toolsets can lead us into the 'God of the Gap' argument, often evoked when science alone is unable to provide us with a suitably satisfactory solution or answer. For example, Intelligent Design theories of creation emerged as an attempt to reconcile the cognitive dissonance evoked when trying to use the quantitative rational mindset (e.g. generating a god to cover the gap); but this attempt is a use of the rational (earth) toolset to address irrational (heaven) questions and thus it is doomed to fail. The existence of God is not a testable (falsifiable) hypothesis. Therefore, do not apply scientific methods to test it.

> *When I am working on a problem, I never think about beauty but when I have finished, if the solution is not beautiful, I know it is wrong.* - Buckminster Fuller

But yes, we still do pull God in to cover over our gaps, ... and our gasps! Often we are too awed to solely rely on a 'Spock-like' objectivity for our judgments and decisions. And thus, the 'God of Gasp' specter is raised.

But so what? Was not Einstein, the math genius and visionary, also most mystical?

> *Theoretical physicists accept the need for mathematical beauty as an act of faith ... For example, the main reason why the theory of relativity is so universally accepted is its mathematical beauty.* - Paul A. M. Dirac

And similarly, the 'nonquantitatives' among us often hold mathematics and quantitation in 'awe' and are easily swayed and deceived by numbers (their own God of Gasp, perhaps?). Quantitative methods can have a real power for some, especially those not well-versed in math and data analysis. Examples include Lyme disease where fervent conviction leads to aggressively testing for parasites, hoping to explain and objectively diagnosis chronic and vague symptoms. Another potent power comes with the looking at visual tests such as spinal MRI scans for back pain. Even some Heaven Helpers like to push forth pseudosciences like crystal vibrations, energy fields, auras, and extrasensory powers, often in an attempt to gain acceptance in the science-based world of healthcare. But there really is no need to chase crazy theories. Belief is powerful, and is enough. Phenomenonalistic, individualistic, pragmatism à la William James, is the proper approach.

> *Our esteem for facts has not neutralized in us all religiousness. It is itself almost religious. Our scientific temper is devout.* - William James

According to Pragmatism, the truth of an idea can never be proven. William James directed us to focus on its usefulness. He disliked structuralism's breaking down mental events into their smallest elements. Instead, he embraced the wholeness of an event, taking into account the environment's impact on behavior.

> *The test of the machine is the satisfaction it gives you. There isn't any other test. If the machine produces tranquility it's right. If it disturbs you it's wrong until either the machine or your mind is changed.* - Robert M. Pirsig

But how can it work? What is going on? Here we turn to heaven's tools in order to bridge over the 'gaps' and 'gasps' remaining after applying earth tools to our endeavors.

Laura Kragie, MD: Be the Rainbow • Bridge Heaven and Earth

HEAVEN

I label the areas not easily provable or described by our earthy scientific methods, as 'Heaven.' And Jung is most adept in handling these types of topics. Carl Gustav Jung was a physician, anthropologist, archeologist, early neuroscientist and psychiatrist. Today's Myers Briggs personality profile test is based on his description and analysis of personality components. He dedicated most of his lifework, though, to understanding the unconscious aspects of our minds, being most famous for using the Interpretation of Dreams to probe it. Your "unconscious" peripheral mind is one of heaven's greatest tools.

If your rational conscious mind is most like the fovea of your retina, the central area of keenest vision, then the unconscious (or subconscious) mind is then more like your peripheral vision. Holograms are contained there, i.e. the huge multitude of sensory input and analysis performed outside the conscious-aware main focus of your mind. Even without your conscious will or direction, you mentally create a 360 degree subliminal image of events, thoughts, imaginings, and memories. If you can somehow get into your own 'mind's eye' then you could view all, from various perspectives — physical, emotional, spiritual — just as if you were viewing the sparkling rainbows of light refracted from all the many facets of an emerald cut diamond.

The peripheral mind acts as does the Pointillism approach to image formation — it connects the sensory dots. The artist George Seurat used Pointillism to show that it is the mind that combines and assembles an image evoked from discrete points. His tiny juxtaposed dots of multicolored paint allow his viewer to blend colors optically in their own mind, rather than having the colors physically blended in the pigment painted on the picture canvas.

> *Words ... do not seem to play any role in my mechanism of thought. The physical entities which seem to serve as elements in thought are certain signs and more or less clear images which can be 'voluntarily' reproduced and combined ... before there is any connection with logical construction in words or other signs ... These physical entities are of visual and some of muscular type.* - Albert Einstein

Another analogy helpful for understanding the workings of your peripheral mind, is the concept of Embodiment. Meanings arise from and are conditioned by the patterns of our own bodily experiences. Philosophies that separate mind from body, cognition from emotion, and logic from wonder, are incomplete because imagination links your cognitive and bodily functions. Images, qualities, emotions, and metaphors are all connected to your physical encounters with the world. All are fundamentally derived from your senses. This shows up strongly in linguistics, the study of language, where they describe 'conceptual metaphors.' These emerge as early as infancy and involve space, time, moving, controlling, and other experiences of the body. Our daily language is chock full of these body-based metaphors, like 'push the idea through' or it is going to be a 'rough day.' Brain scans show that you actually mentally sense a rough texture when you say or read that metaphor, even though you may be just referring to a difficult work day and not literally, a sandpaper-filled day. And just by clenching your muscles you can activate willpower, facilitating self-control, when facing a challenge.

> *Language is the amber in which a thousand precious and subtle thoughts have been safely embedded and preserved.* - Richard C. Trench

In a similar vein, William James proposed that an external event triggers a physiological reaction in us, which we then interpret; emotions are then 'caused' by our mind's interpretations of these physiological reactions. Physical sensations 'feedback' from our own bodies and tell our minds what emotions we are 'feeling.' This cycle of body sensation leading to mind interpretation, is another kind of Pointillism — of emotions — the interpretation of discrete, discernable sensations coalescing into an 'emotional state.' The most familiar of these is the 'Fight or Flight' response to stressors. Feel the adrenaline first, then identify it as being a state of 'fear.'

> *We don't laugh because we're happy — we're happy because we laugh.* - William James

Did you know that your facial expressions indicating your emotions are similar to those in other human cultures and therefore are universal? Actually, your face doesn't just show your emotions, it controls your emotions. Facial expressions have a role in how your own emotions develop inside of you, not only in how you display them for others to see. When we are happy, we smile, yes? Even more true, is that when we smile, we 'become' happy. Trying to get rid of your depression? First thing, start smiling. And do not botox your smiling eyes away. People injected with the toxin actually end up with diminished emotional intensity to display on their face, and less intensity to feel.

Women who botox their faces are less able to read emotional expressions on other people's faces. So maybe related, too, is the fact that physically following and imitating others folks' facial expressions can help you to experience empathy, i.e. shared emotions. We also respond to expressions and gestures from others folks' bodies, and these feed back and play into our own emotions — the well-known concept of mirroring. Perhaps this is the basis for that cliché, 'monkey see, monkey do;' and maybe after a few back and forth cycles, it turns into, 'birds of a feather, flock together.' Yawning is a good example. When a person yawns, those around him start yawning. Well, that yawn transmission happens sooner and more often, between close friends, relatives and mates — those we empathize with — than among strangers. This emotional empathy also enables us to picture ourselves living as the characters do when we read fiction; brain scans show us internalizing and mirroring in ourselves, whatever the novel's protagonist experiences.

Sometimes we can use an actual physical mirror image of a limb to simulate bodily feedback in order to lessen phantom limb pain. Referring again to the concept of Embodiment, the 'feel' of your body is reproduced as an image in your mind. The visual sight of the mirror image of your healthy limb triggers your memories of healthier times with it, and these mental images can sometimes override and correct the confused phantom image of the missing, yet hurting, limb.

Our enigmatic peripheral mind also seems to be wired to 'want to believe' in things. Our brains are belief filters, busily seeking out patterns from the sensory data flooding into it. And these patterns are then connected to meaning and ideas. Remember the 'Fight or Flight' scenario? Well, similar to William James' view of emotions and reflexes, beliefs come first and our explanations for those beliefs, then follow. Just as viewing a Pointillistic Seurat painting forms an image out of the painted colored dots, our brains connect the sensory dots of our world into meaningful patterns that explain why things happen; these patterns then become our beliefs. Once beliefs get formed in our brain, we tend to seek and find evidence to confirm these previously determined convictions.

And this is just fine with our man, William James. He embraced subjective, spiritual experiences. He disliked a "medical materialism that finishes St. Paul by calling his vision on the road to Damascus as a discharging lesion of the occipital cortex" and "snuffs out St. Theresa as a hysteric." James' advice is simple and direct: believe, if one wishes, based on faith, that is, without requiring proof or evidence.

> *The most beautiful experience we can have is the mysterious.* - Albert Einstein

Not just in dreams, but Carl Gustav Jung also elucidated the mind's capacity for Magical Thinking — a state of mind that is not grounded in clear cut cause and effect, but instead is tinged with mysticism and fantasy. Magical thinking weights and links coincidences pulled from our real world. Our brains will leap to connect unrelated events and coincidences because it is the master at finding patterns in all things, but not so good at discerning the actual type of relation between those events — causal? random? correlative? As adults, we retain our desire for indulging in the Magical Thinking that was so prominent in our childhoods. It is an essential, primal instinct. Without it, or when suppressing it, it can lead us to abuse psychogenic substances, in a desperate pursuit of reclaiming it. Jung conferred with Bill W. when he was developing his ideas for Alcoholics

Laura Kragie, MD: Be the Rainbow • Bridge Heaven and Earth

Anonymous. Jung also tried to help Sigmund Freud deal with his struggle over cocaine addiction, though apparently without success. Freud was vehemently against all things mystical, despite his lifelong study of the individual's unconscious, and he would not consider the existence of any higher power.

> *The sway of alcohol over mankind is unquestionably due to its power to stimulate the mystical faculties of human nature, usually crushed to earth by the cold facts and dry criticisms of the sober hour.* - William James

So now we know that, our minds embody sensations to create emotions, and wire them together to create beliefs. And we cling to our early instincts of Magical Thinking that allude to the mystical. Well, Jung's study of the Collective Unconscious and his Interpretation of Dreams also brought out the cross-cultural, cross-epochal, concept of Archetypes. These are like story units, composed from complex patterns of belief and emotions, hard-wired in the human brain — e.g. the Hero Archetype. Is this perhaps another form of mental Pointillism, but of icons? Perhaps our minds connect 'hieroglyphic' dots of meaning and emotion to form these? Art is chock full of iconic symbols and archetypes — as the movie *Inception* illustrates. They can trigger choices subliminally, setting off a cascade of ideas and emotions tied to ancient cultural storylines.

> *The mythos is a building of analogues upon analogues upon analogues. These fill the collective consciousness of all communicating mankind. Every last bit of it.* - Robert M. Pirsig

Scientists, too, are desperate to find some kind of magic in their lives; take note of all the science fiction and action heroes that fill out the geek culture. And Heaven Helpers too, are desperate to find the mystery in their lives, as manifested in all those stories containing visions of God. Magic and mystery together form the miracles we seek in life, driven in part by our instinct for Magical Thinking. All of us are trying to get away from boredom and lack of novelty, seeking distraction from pain or lack of pleasure. This Magical Thinking instinct is intense, strong, and pervasive.

> *Science without religion is lame, religion without science is blind.* - Albert Einstein

THE HEAVENLY TOOLSET

In this world, there are many different practices and practitioners, using something other than hard scientific methods for their healing. This is not the place, nor the time, to evaluate each. Instead, here I describe some of the components that perhaps, may be involved in the positive actions and effects of Heaven Helpers.

> *Like a bridge over troubled water, I will ease your mind.* - Paul Simon

ATTITUDES of MIND

Motivation, Inspiration: Use your anger, determination, and survival instinct to 'fire up' your engines. Fight cancer. Conquer addiction. Squelch fear. Competing with yourself and with others can help you reach towards your personal best in performance. If you clench your fists and set your jaw, you can actually increase the strength of your willpower; and yes, it's due to the process of Embodiment. Think of your heroes, too ... and imagine being them.

> *A person who has not passed through the inferno of their passions has never overcome them.* - Carl Jung

Gratitude: One of the most well known practices espoused by the Heaven Helpers to increase happiness and decrease depressive symptoms is the Three Blessings exercise. Each night before going to bed you write down three good things that happened to you during that particular day. It is a variation of the childhood routine of bedtime prayers, thanking God for loved ones and the day's blessings. It works even better if you can vary the times and topics of the exercise; keeps it from going stale.

> *The greatest discovery of my generation is that human beings can alter their lives by altering their attitudes of mind.* - William James

Humor: "Laughter is the best medicine," says **Readers Digest**. Laughter stimulates many organs. Laughter enhances your intake of oxygen-rich air, stimulates your heart, lungs and muscles, and increases the endorphins released by your brain. It activates and relieves your stress. A full-hearted LMAO laugh fires you up and then cools you down, leaving you relaxed. Laughter can also break the pain-spasm cycle of muscle disorders. Maybe, too, good humor can lead to stronger hearts; people suffering from heart disease were less likely to respond with a laugh when compared to similar folks without heart disease. Patients are both more tolerant of pain, and require less medication, after watching a comedy. But note, the benefits from the movie only come if you control what it is you want to watch, not have it assigned to you. It soothes tension. Laughter can also stimulate circulation and aid muscle relaxation. And humor is infectious. The sound of roaring laughter is contagious; when laughter is shared, it binds people together and increases shared happiness and intimacy.

> *Common sense and a sense of humor are the same thing, moving at different speeds. A sense of humor is just common sense, dancing.* - William James

Optimism, Positive Mental Attitude (PMA): Optimism versus pessimism was compared in brain scans of the posterior parietal cortex, where sensory stimuli are transformed into movement plans. The posterior parietal cortex performance was affected by the subjects' belief of success or failure. Our belief in our likely success or failure at a given task and its consequences directly affects the amount of neural effort we put forth in these movement-planning motor circuits.

When we have a positive hopeful confidence we will expend our energy and willpower to go into that holographic peripheral mindspace to find the creative solution to our dilemmas. Such is the core philosophy underlying the popular 'Law of Attraction' and PMA movements. What is your desired outcome? What is your goal? What determines a 'success' for you? Which phenomenon is desired? Longevity, prolongation of life? Or do you seek being at peace, serene, pain free, calm, content? Or motivated, energized, activated? Use your anger to conquer cancer. Visualize and feel what you want to have happen. It's important to use your imagination and see yourself as fit and well, to become well.

> *If you want to build a ship, don't drum up people together to collect wood and don't assign them tasks and work, but rather teach them to long for the endless immensity of the sea.* - Antoine de Saint-Exupery

Believe in good outcome … or believe in bad outcome? Remember the Hmong tribe from Laos who suffered sudden death episodes arising from their fear of bad spirits, when they immigrated to the USA, away from their rural Asian villages? And remember those brain-imaging studies from the pain and placebo trials that identified an expectation pathway in our brains? Patients whose prefrontal cortex (the decision-making executive part of brains) lit up when anticipating pain relief, felt less pain. Self-Fulfilling Prophecy — it really means, 'you land where you look.' So, decide to look up!

> *Talk unbelief, and you will have unbelief; but talk faith, and you will have faith. According to the seed sown will be the harvest.* - Ellen G. White

MEDITATION and SLEEP

Beauty is something we are driven to seek, in nature, in faces, even in math. It can induce awe and mysticism, as well as peace and serenity. A most popular resource is in the Great Outdoors amidst Mother Nature; think of Thoreau's discourse on Walden Pond. Double rainbows are pretty awesome, too :-) And of course, for many males their choice meditation is hunting or fishing; yes their real reason for safari is to commune with the landscape more than chasing and killing its inhabitants. Meditation with nature is just as much a part of a hunter's psyche as it is with liberal environmentalists. For those in crowded urban spaces, carefully-structured Japanese Zen Gardens are designed to induce happiness and contentment, even within the concrete jungle.

> *The true harvest of my daily life is somewhat as intangible and indescribable as the tints of morning or evening. It is a little star-dust caught, a segment of the rainbow which I have clutched.* - Henry David Thoreau

But when we are without an external place to seek it, we are then guided to imagine our own Inner Landscape of Beauty — told to "go to your peaceful place" and find that inner Garden of Eden, our own Paradise. To help us with building this interior state of calm, we can perhaps turn to watching fish for our meditation. Gazing, for real or video, at aquarium fish reduces stress, lowers blood pressure, calms hyperactive children and even lessens the need for pain meds in dental patients. And for those of you on the go, yes, there is an app for that - 'The Koi Pond.'

Meditation induces a set of integrated physiologic changes termed, the Relaxation Response. Many decades ago, Herbert Benson M.D. described the Relaxation Response, which is the opposite of the stress response. He determined for us, the basic fundamental components necessary to induce a drop in oxygen consumption, heart rate, pressure, and respiratory rate. First, we need to adopt a "let it happen" attitude. To shift the mind from logical, externally oriented thought, we should have a constant repetitive stimulus: a sound, word, or phrase repeated silently or aloud; or fixing your gaze at an object. Attending to the normal rhythm of our own breathing amplifies the repetition of sound or word. Your deep rhythmic breathing induces a parasympathetic-like state, counteracting any residual sympathetic 'fight or flight' state. You may also find these fundamental components in the repetitive cadence from jogging, marching, horseback riding, rocking in a chair, rocking a baby, the pendulum of swinging, or baby bouncing in a chair. Knitting and crocheting too, induces such a Zen state, in addition to focus, patience and social support.

Meditations can induce 'twilight' states that seem to impart benefits similar to a nap. Sleep states are restorative, giving escape and relief. The lack of sleep, insomnia, ranks up there with chronic pain as one of our major health burdens. Our total well-being deteriorates without adequate sleep. It is a crucial biomarker in any measure of therapeutic effect and quality of life. And this involves not just hours asleep, but quality of sleep and whether the phases of sleep achieve their normal cycling through REM and nonREM phases.

> *Those who look outwards, dream, but those who look inwards, awake.* - Carl Jung

Sleep's REM state and its dreams, serve to process thoughts and emotions and to form memories. A night's sleep protects memories from the day, including your emotional reaction to events. If it is a negative event, then staying awake is better, in order to avoid 'solidifying' the bad vibes associated with it. Using Lucid Dreaming, as was shown in the movie *Inception*, perhaps we can 'plant' memories in order to edit was is already there. There are some therapists using the game TETRIS to compete with PTSD nightmares. It is only with this REM state recycling, that memories retain their strength, so any ways to re-see and re-write a better story ending, help these patients.

Both Albert Einstein and Thomas Edison deliberately used exercises of self-hypnosis in order to get themselves into a creative state. There is the hynagogic trance state that happens just as you are switching from the conscious awake state and slipping into a REM dream state. If we can learn to capture ourselves in that transition, it can allow us access to subliminal aspects in our peripheral brain. We have used these types of hypnosis to assist folks in coping with their traumas or in kicking an addictive habit, allowing them to set intentions to quit and relieve the stressors driving addictions.

> *No problem can be solved from the same level of consciousness that created it.* - Albert Einstein

Alpha waves are a signal in the brain that correlates with states of pre-sleep relaxation. And when we are relaxed, we are more likely to have those big 'aha!' moments of insight where our impossible problems get solved. So how do we find some way to relax and get those alpha waves? We could practice meditation techniques, but we can also use binaural beats — a unique audio technology — to induce twilight states. (And yes, there is an app for that.) Within just minutes, it synchronizes your brainwaves down to the alpha and theta frequencies, the ones best for inducing lucid dreams through the hypnagogic state. In order to take advantage of your hypnagogia to capture your creativity, you do need to keep a certain degree of conscious cognitive awareness as your physical body is drifting off to sleep. It does come with practice, though.

Brain scans of experienced meditators show that they can prevent their minds from wandering; they are able to turn down activity in areas of the brain that are usually seen as up-regulated in anxiety states, and in those folks with attention deficit hyperactivity disorder, autism and schizophrenia. Meditators have decreased activity in the default mode network (which consists of the medial prefrontal and posterior cingulate cortex) and increased activity in those regions associated with our self-monitoring and cognitive control. They seemed to have developed a default mode that is more in the present moment and less centered on self. Positive changes extend, as well, to their immune system. For example, they develop more robust responses to a flu virus challenge, than the nonmeditators.

And serious intense yogic practices can have a direct impact on the heart. Experienced practitioners can even become consciously aware of their own heart rate and blood pressure fluctuations, and even modulate them. Nidra yoga practitioners gain restorative rest and improved sleep, coinciding with increases in brain dopamine.

SPIRITUALITY, FAITH, BELIEF and PRAYER

Light can penetrate dark, but dark can't penetrate light. - Kryon

"Opium of the masses," Marx's description of religion, may actually be true, though not in the way he may have supposed. There is the classic Relaxation Response, and that does occur with prayer; it consists of slowed focused breathing, reduction in blood pressure and heart rate, reduction in anxiety, and a sense of serenity. A spectrum of many different types of prayer practices can elicit the Relaxation Response, just by using the common themes of repetitive movement and speaking / breathing. Examples include:

- Bowing and rocking your body, as seen with Muslim or Jewish prayer rituals

- Dizzying trance-like twirls of the whirling dervishes

- Repetitive prayers, mantras or affirmations, such as with saying the rosary or Gregorian chants

The God Brain: Scientists have found that the brains of people who spend many hours in prayer and meditation are somewhat different. They have those slow, large-amplitude delta waves, typical of a person in intense meditation or deep sleep, yet they are awake. And when they are meditating, their frontal lobes light up, but their parietal lobes dim down. This parietal area is where we have our sensory information center, orienting us to 'self' and 'outside self.' These folks report feeling as if there is a loss of their sense of self as an individual, and blurring the boundary between self and others. They describe feeling a sense of a higher, larger power.

A human being is a part of a whole, called by us 'universe', a part limited in time and space. He experiences himself, his thoughts and feelings as something separated from the rest... a kind of optical delusion of his consciousness. This delusion is a kind of prison for us, restricting us to our personal desires and to

Laura Kragie, MD: Be the Rainbow • Bridge Heaven and Earth

> *affection for a few persons nearest to us. Our task must be to free ourselves from this prison by widening our circle of compassion to embrace all living creatures and the whole of nature in its beauty.* -Albert Einstein

They also looked at brains of people who claim to have active numinous spiritual experiences. Some subjects, who reported visions of God, showed fired up temporal lobes, a part of the limbic system of the old reptile brain. This system handles not just sound, smell and some vision but also memory and especially emotion. In one woman who claimed to channel God and speak in tongues, they found that her brain — unlike the brains of the meditators — had diminished activity in her frontal lobes and her parietal lobes were lit up. It looked as if her brain was having an internal one-on-one dialogue with God.

The Belief Brain: Scientists scanned brains of volunteers while they responded to assertions relating to math and ethics. The statements that were consistent with the subjects' own personal beliefs, lit up the ventral medial prefrontal cortex, the brain region known for processing reward, emotion and taste; these assertions made them feel good. Areas associated with taste, pain and disgust lit up when the statements induced their disbelief; these assertions made them feel bad.

So ... are we experiencing 'God' in those neuronal networks or are we just inherently prepped for any 'encounter' with something sacred? Does either explanation even matter, if the experience leads us to an improved state of mind and body? In patients with HIV, those who turned to God after their diagnosis maintained a lower viral load and sustained their levels of immune cells at a much higher rate than those who turned away from God. Conversely, those patients who felt abandoned by God, deteriorated much faster.

> *Spiritual energy flows in and produces effects in the phenomenal world.* - William James

Perhaps that nonverbal and verbal communication concept, Embodiment, parallels the biblical story of Jesus Christ — he sought physical corporal embodiment. This literally means dropping fully into one's body, seeking physical expression. Is this then, the phenomenon of 'being born again'? Spiritual rebirth? Reincarnation? Seeking self-actualization? Well, heaven's tools can lead you to feel very open to the messages of the world around you, as clues come through to show you how to go about embodying new experiences and sensations into your psyche. So do be careful and be aware of who and what you hang out with ... may it be more like a Gandhi and not a Hitler. Or, perhaps even ... more like a Rumi and not a Bin Laden.

> *Faith is much better than belief. Belief is when someone else does the thinking.*
> -Buckminster Fuller

POWER of TOUCH

Laying on of Hands, Doctor to Patient, Priest to Soul: Humankind was truly given a profound legacy in Hands-On Healing. The laying on of hands is a religious ritual that accompanies certain religious practices, which are found throughout the world in varying forms. It was practiced by many cultures for thousands of years. In Greek mythology you find Chiron, the wounded healer Centaur, teaching Asclepius, the God of Medicine, the power of touch to heal. In Christian churches, this touching with the hands is used during sacraments, healing services, and blessings, to invoke the Holy Spirit.

> *A woman was bowed down with a spirit of Infirmity, and Jesus laid hands on her, and healed her.* - Luke 13:11, 13

> *he who believes in me will also do the works that I do; and greater works than these will he do.* - Jesus, to his disciples in John 14:12

Human to human connections start with touch. One of the most basic ways to establish trust is to touch. Babies are calmed by swaddling ... the feel of being held and embraced. And adults are really just big babies, especially when hurting and vulnerable. Mata Amritanandamayi Devi, the hugging saint, administers her charity and blessings with warm embraces of her following. And with athletes, the more they high-five or hug their own teammates, the better they perform their game. Folks facing stressful tasks, lower their blood pressure and heart rate if they hold hands or were hug.

> *One touch is worth 10,000 words.* - Harold Bloomfield

Hand-holding or hugging decreases the stress hormone cortisol. In addition to calming us down and reducing our stress response, a friendly touch can also release the neuropeptide oxytocin, which is also involved in the bonding of mother to baby during breastfeeding. It is associated with our feelings of devotion and trust; a cuddle hormone. Oxytocin levels elevate especially after we receive a therapeutic massage.

Being touched can be pleasant. Brain scan studies show that the orbital frontal cortex becomes activated in response to friendly touch. Yes this is the same area that responds to sweet tastes and pleasing smells, and touch is a powerful rewarding stimulus. There is a class of nerve fibers in the skin that specifically sends the brain pleasure messages, when stroked at a certain speed, about 4-5 cm per second. Having a massage after strenuous exercise not only feels good, it reduces inflammation in muscles at the cellular level. Many people find that having a massage after exercise reduces their muscle pain, similar to taking anti-inflammatory drugs. And deep tissue massage can decrease the neuropeptide hormone arginine vasopressin, which constricts blood vessels and raises blood pressure.

Most intriguing is the phenomenon where touching your own hand can reduce pain from a burn; simple self-touch can minimize complex central pain. This was illustrated using the thermal-grill sensory illusion. When subjects are asked to touch a very warm object and then, right afterward, touch a cool or room-temperature object, the subjects' brains fool them into believing that the second object feels excruciatingly hot, even though nothing has happened to their flesh. That burning sensation is actually central (brain) pain. In the experiment, participants immersed their index and ring fingers in hot water and their middle fingers in tepid water. Those middle fingers seemed to be painfully hotter than they actually were. The scientists then had participants repeat the experiment with only their right fingers. Then immediately after, the subjects used the same three fingers on their left hand to now touch the wet fingers on the right immersed hand. This mere touch from the noninvolved, nonpainful hand took away that burning pain sensation in that immersed right hand!

For back pain patients, getting lessons in the Alexander Technique has longterm benefits, and may be even more effective than massage or exercise. The Alexander Technique is a form of bodywork that educates its pupils into consciously using their bodies more efficiently in their routine movements. It works by bringing unconscious habits up to conscious critical reflection so that they can be worked on, making their pupils more cognizant of their 'faulty sensory awareness.' Pupils learn to differentiate aspects of their movement in such activities as standing and sitting from a chair. The Alexander teacher uses their hands and touch to adjust and convey the sense of the work and how the body / self is to be aligned. Conscious control is most important. "Re-education is not a process of adding something, but of restoring something. It was to meet the need of restoring actual conditions of use and functioning which had been previously experienced and afterwards lost, that my technique for the re-education of the use of the self was evolved." - Frederick Alexander

> *I know of no more encouraging fact than the unquestionable ability of man to elevate his life by conscious behavior.* - Henry David Thoreau

PETS

Pet Therapy: here come the cute and cuddly heaven helpers, the Animal Therapists. Yes, indeed, our furry best friends contribute mightily to the healing professions. Petting zoos are a staple guaranteed to provide endless entertainment for kids and their adult caretakers. It continues into adulthood, where puppies brought in from the shelters help college student's deal with stress of their final exams. Pets are mood enhancing and help lessen depression in AIDS patients. And they lessen hypertension in stockbrokers who walk dogs and play fetch with them. Having a pet facilitates rehabilitation and survivorship after a heart attack. And those who own pets — yes, they do out-live folks without them.

Pet therapy added to help recovery from total joint-replacement surgery leads to less need for pain medication. One dog breed in particular, the Xoloitzcuintli (Mexican Hairless), acts like a live heating pad placed on the site of pain. The animals are a source of encouragement and are great motivators of chronic pain sufferers, pushing them to stay more active.

> *My little old dog: a heart-beat at my feet.* - Edith Wharton

Society of Friends ran a retreat for the mentally ill where patients learned to care for animals and work in a gardens as part of their rehab therapy. Delta Society registers "Pet Partners" and these include rabbits, guinea pigs, cats, goats, pot-bellied pigs, horses, donkeys, parrots, cockatoos, chickens, and llamas. But dogs are by far the most common and popular animal therapists. Specialty trained service dogs are essential assists to the disabled, the autistic, and the epileptic. Cerebral palsy individuals benefit from kitten therapy. Cats provide that essential component, touch, especially when they crawl up into your lap so you can pet them. Picking up and interacting with these cuddly balls of fur, helps these patients improve their motor and sensory skills.

A returning wounded warrior launched Pets to Vets, a nonprofit group that links service members and first responders with shelter animals, and helps them with the expenses and training. Pound dogs soothe emotionally wounded warriors with their companionship and unconditional support.

> *No one appreciates the very special genius of your conversation as a dog does.* - Christopher Morley

Pets help with social support. When out walking, having a dog with us can make us more approachable (puppies are especially good 'chick magnets'). It gives neighbors a reason to stop and talk, thereby increasing the number of people to meet, providing an opportunity to increase our network of friends and acquaintances. Nursing home residents reported less loneliness during time spent visiting with dogs, than when they spent time with other people! All these benefits can reduce the amount of stress people experience when socially isolated and without social support from others.

> *If you want a friend in Washington, get a dog.* - Harry Truman

Therapeutic horseback riding is an emerging field where horses are used as a tool for physical therapy, emotional growth and learning. They assist those disabled from amputation, cerebral palsy, autism, MS, and stroke. Because horseback riding's cadence can gently and rhythmically move the rider's body in a manner similar to a human gait, riders with physical disabilities improve in flexibility, balance and muscle strength. As a result of these lessons, poise, posture, strength and flexibility improve. Many riders experience an emotional connection to their horse. The unique relationship formed with your horse can lead to increased confidence, patience and self-esteem. For those riders who cannot walk, their horse becomes their vehicle of transport, and thus greatly expanding their effective universe.

Laura Kragie, MD: Be the Rainbow • Bridge Heaven and Earth

MUSIC, DANCE and SINGING

> *I think music in itself is healing. It's an explosive expression of humanity. It's something we are all touched by.* - Billy Joel

Emotionally intense music releases dopamine in those pleasure and reward centers of the brain, just like food, sex and drugs does. Autonomic responses such as goose bumps correlate with the amount of dopamine released, even when the evocative music is sad. So, the more intensely emotional a song is, the more we crave that song. An example is the recent Grammy winner, Adele's "Someone Like You." It features an appoggiatura, which is an ornamental note that clashes with the melody, only enough to create a dissonant sound, generating tension in the listener. When the music returns back to the anticipated melody, then the tension resolves, and that feels good to the listener. That's when listeners get their goose bumps, at these moments of resolution.

But music in our brains is never standing alone. Scans show that while listening to songs and instrumentals, we are imagining moving our bodies along with the melody and rhythm. So, yes, all us can dance ... at least in our mind's eye.

> *And we should consider every day lost on which we have not danced at least once.* - Friedrich Nietzsche

The Persian, Jalaluddin Rumi (1207–1273) was a poet, mystic, and founder of the Whirling Dervishes of Sufism. He established the Dervishes to help us reach the rapture state where we dissolve into love, sacrificing our mind to love. It is a complete submission, unity, and annihilation of self, into the Beloved. This is the state that is known as *nirvana* in Buddhism and as *fana fillah* in Islam. The Sema ritual of the Dervishes shows that everything revolves. The Whirling Dervish intentionally and consciously participates in the shared revolution of all other beings. Through turning movement, body posturing, mental focus, and sound, the Dervish achieves ecstasy through a union with God. This dance trance ceremony represents the human being's spiritual journey, an ascent by means of intelligence and love into Perfection.

Laura Kragie, MD: Be the Rainbow • Bridge Heaven and Earth

Whosoever knoweth the power of the dance, dwelleth in God. - Jalaluddin Rumi

Whirling dance, African drumming, hearing binaural beats of select sound frequencies — all can induce a trance state, and ultimately better sleep, focus, relaxation, and dream states. Humming that creates a vibration in the chest, self-soothes and calms you when you are anxious and afraid. It is a connection to your limbic emotional brain, and eases pain. And in people who are deeply disoriented by Alzheimer's or schizophrenia, music can calm and organize their internal chaos.

Music is a safe kind of high. - Jimi Hendrix

Music used as therapy speeds stroke patients' rehabilitation from aphasia. Even when their speech cortex has been damaged and they cannot speak, they can still sing. Rep. Gabby Giffords course of recovery from her brain trauma provides a current example of the benefit of Melodic Intonation Therapy, where all conversational words are sung. Music and song help autistics learn to communicate too. During recovery from depression and loss, music can actually feel like it is 'piercing the heart' when it suddenly connects, releasing the frozen grief and restoring enthusiasm for life. And, of course, a great bouncy dance tune, gets Parkinsonian patients up and moving, when nothing else can.

Music's the medicine of the mind. - John A. Logan

Music therapy combined with relaxation imagery can reduce patients' pain and nausea felt after bone marrow transplant. It is difficult and expensive to perform RCT testing music treatments, but some animal studies do provide some insights. In research experiments with mice given heart transplants from an unrelated donor, the time to rejection was measured. For a week following the operation, the mice continuously listened to Verdi's opera *La Traviata*, a selection of Mozart concertos, music by Enya, or a range of single monotones. The mice that listened to opera lived longest, with those who listened to Mozart next, then Enya, and the monotone group the shortest. And the music did not work on deaf mice — they lived only as long as the monotones group.

Laura Kragie, MD: Be the Rainbow • Bridge Heaven and Earth

Songbirds, the first robins signaling the return of spring after a long winter, bring us a sense of joy. Studies have found that bird songs make traffic noise more tolerable, make people feel less crowded and can even influence circadian rhythms. Birdsong has healing effects; surgery patients needed less pain relief and were far more relaxed when exposed to birds singing. For ancient seafaring sailors, song birds were signs of tremendous relief for they signified that land was near. In the myth of the great flood, Noah and those on his ark heard the birds sing and knew that land was finally re-emerging. It coincided with the appearance of the rainbow. It's not surprising that novelist Suzanne Collins chose to use a song bird as her underlying symbol throughout her best selling **Hunger Games** trilogy.

Parrots are considered the most intelligent of birds. They are able to mimic human speech, and some are able to associate words with their meanings and form simple sentences. They are expressive companions who provide social comfort and support. And they too, like to hum to self-soothe, and so doing, soothe us.

> *Music is the universal language of mankind.* - Henry Wadsworth Longfellow

The origin of speech is social, it requires the interaction of mother and infant. A baby learns to distinguish sounds for spoken language by first listening to their mother's cooing and baby talk. And music lies beneath spoken language, especially Motherese and lullabies. This universal speech — the slow, exaggerated, singsong intonation — is used by all mothers of all cultures, all languages. The lullaby mutually calms mother and child, because its regular rhythmic breathing and slow steady cadence relax muscles and lower heart rate.

Music is the social superglue, bonding us. Synchronous, coordinated song and movement are fundamental to creating strong cohesion amongst group members. Singing together with others stimulates release of the neuropeptide oxytocin, helping to forge connections. Singing together can seem to create a sense of collective consciousness, larger than the single self. The Hallelujah chorus sung in church at Easter can provide this kind of group emotive expressive outlet. Music can also motivate and encourage, especially if done in social groups. 'Call and response' music and song is found across cultures and epochs. We see it in gospel choirs, chain gangs, marching soldiers, cheerleader squads, and marching bands. Nothing beats its ability to synchronize and energize.

> *Music expresses that which cannot be said and on which it is impossible to be silent.* -Victor Hugo

PLAY, EXERCISE and SPORTS

Exercise releases muscle tension and stiffness and is another form of relaxation and pain-reduction. Regular exercise guards against migraine headaches. It can work as well as medication or relaxation techniques in preventing these attacks. It even helps offset symptoms of menopause. A good workout improves sleep quality. Running, swimming, swinging, riding and baby chair bouncing all have that repetitive cadence — perhaps inducing Benson's Relaxation Response?

> *Let the beauty we love be what we do.* - Jalaluddin Rumi

Yoga practices focus on learning physical poses, which are called asanas, and usually include some form of breathing technique and a meditation. Yoga asanas induce changes in your breathing, emphasizing the deepening and lengthening your breath. This stimulates Benson's Relaxation Response. It elevates mood, relieves anxiety, lessens pain, and increases confidence, motivation. As it relates to the Embodiment concept, your body feels powerful, strong, free, confident, and this feeds back into your mind as a relaxed optimistic state. Firm muscles can firm willpower. The series of yoga poses work by safely stretching your muscles, clearing the build up of lactic acid, and thus releasing your stiffness, tension, pain, and fatigue. Yoga increases your range of joint motion and gives you a greater sense of ease and fluidity throughout your body. It also can change your emotional limbic brain, reducing the activity in the fear-generating amygdala.

Aerobic exercise is a first line treatment for many physical and mental illnesses and its use with unipolar depression has antianxiolytic properties. Psychiatric patients taking antipsychotics are at risk of metabolic syndrome, and this does respond to exercise. Some health benefits arising from yoga practice include more flexibility, strength, and balance; reduced symptoms of post-traumatic stress, including rage, insomnia and anxiety. On top of all that, regular exercise may even reduce your risk of breast, colon, and possibly prostate cancers.

> *Of all human powers operating on the affairs of mankind, none is greater than that of competition.* - Henry Clay

Downhill skiing, skate boarding, surfing, speed skating — all can give you that most awesome adrenaline rush, a feeling of being totally alive. This is the good aspect of your 'fight or flight' response. When releasing adrenaline, you also release dopamine, which acts as a natural painkiller. And with activation of your dopamine reward center you are mentally and physically motivated to perform at peak. It causes your muscles respire faster, improving your strength and speed. The satisfaction from a good workout probably also involves dopamine, and makes people want to repeat enjoyable experiences. And then again, too, there are those wonderful endogenous opioids kicking in their part to the party.

> *Live daringly, boldly, fearlessly. Taste the relish to be found in competition — in having put forth the best within you.* - Henry J. Kaiser

Playing with children is the quickest way for you to access your own inner child. The laughter and spontaneity distracts us away from our own worries, illness, disability and pain. It increases your confidence in taking risks, and coloring outside the lines. As with children, pets are also great at bringing about play, and kids plus pets are truly the most engaging of all.

> *The dog was created especially for children. He is the god of frolic.* - Henry Ward Beecher

And yes, don't forget, we do have apps for all that — e.g. yoga, aerobic workouts, online gaming, and of course, Nintendo Wii.

SOCIAL SUPPORTS

If you do something nice for someone else, doesn't it feel good? So, it shouldn't surprise you to find that practicing random acts of kindness is therapeutic for mood disorders like depression. Positive activity interventions serve as effective, low-cost help for depression. Social ties truly can influence our well-being.

Laura Kragie, MD: Be the Rainbow • Bridge Heaven and Earth

The bird a nest, the spider a web, man friendship. - William Blake

There are many ways people relate to other people — spouses, family, friends, groups — and many ways people are affected by their own social networks. The diversity and multitude of your social connections can directly impact on your health, happiness, and longevity. The plurality of your peeps, affects your overall mortality, incidence of cardiovascular disease, recovery rates, progress of cancer and late life cognition.

Benefits emerge from things like social integration — getting introduced to new events, trends, and experiences beyond those that usually involve you. Think about all those things your teenage kids brought into your life while they were growing up; music, sports, school events, fundraisers. And your own network provides you with opportunities extended to you from your other members; e.g. job referrals, blind dates. Most of all, social networks can insulate or buffer you from the tough times of life. Having people who 'have your back' really helps protect you in times of personal stress. Hopefully, your posse is more like fellow churchgoers rather than gang members, but both can serve that same crucial function.

A man's growth is seen in the successive choirs of his friends. - Ralph Waldo Emerson

Groups socially express their emotions — they sing, dance, and commiserate together, in the pub 'where everyone knows your name.' Humor helps you keep a positive, optimistic outlook through disappointments, and laughing with others is more powerful than laughing alone. Team sports — both as participant and as spectator — allows you to become one with your team, 'willing' them to a win. Friday Night Football in Texas and Baseball in Boston are often described as a religion; the fans fervently identify with their cherished team and empathize with all the other fans as one group. There is a fusion of their emotions with the team's and this extends even out into the online time sphere of Facebook and Twitter. Even a state of limerence emerges in those soldiers participating in military drills where they march in formation — triggering the Relaxation Response plus social bonding — thus cementing the comrades' group loyalty and fidelity.

Coaching from your own health team can serve up the same bennies. Use your group's encouragement and PMA; remember that it can be a self-fulfilling prophecy. A cogent example of this is a saying taken from equestrians riding and jumping horses, "you land where you look." Supportive expressive group therapy, found commonly in mental health practices, emphasizes the sense that you are not alone in your struggle. Patient support groups are all over the internet now, and these groups help each other with suggestions for symptom relief, doctor referrals, as well as providing a place to vent and journal their stories of dealing with disease.

When it comes to beating addiction, no 'therapy' tops the 12 Step Programs. Their social support, as well as spirituality (as a higher power), mediates Alcoholic Anonymous' effectiveness in achieving and maintaining longterm sobriety. Perhaps, connection to God is like being linked-in to the most A-list of social groups. Studies of the brain in those who belong to religious groups show that these type activities engage the same cognitive networks as those involved in social networking. And yes, folks who go to church regularly — whatever faith they have — do live longer. So, if 'birds of a feather flock together'... maybe they are hanging out with the angels?

> *If instead of a gem, or even a flower, we should cast the gift of a loving thought into the heart of a friend, that would be giving as the angels give.* - George MacDonald

FEAR/ INSECURITY / STRESS versus COMFORT / SAFETY / SOOTHED

Fear really amps up pain, anxiety and stress response; all generated in the mind / brain. It fuels and inflames all those nocebo effects. We are put on alert, watching for signs of attack, impending doom. We fear abandonment; fear there will be no rescue from the pain. Aloneness. Solitary confinement truly is our ultimate nonlethal punishment. We turn to God seeking any connection, to any 'other.'

> *The sovereign cure for worry is prayer.* -William James

To get well, to get 'out of our rational heads,' we need to surrender our care into the hands of the healer. Doing so, is very scary, very difficult. To find relief and comfort requires belief and trust.

Laura Kragie, MD: Be the Rainbow • Bridge Heaven and Earth

> *After a heavy storm, a rainbow appears...* - Anon

When sick, we want to feel safe, cared for, back in Mom's embrace, comforted. The Hebrew word for 'mercy' is very similar to their word for 'womb.' Yes, mercy is like the mother's love and protection, in a womb. We need to be soothed. When calmed, your vital energy is no longer being sucked down into that black hole filled with your demons. But it involves letting go — of the negativity, the burdens. To Just Be.

> *The world we see that seems so insane is the result of a belief system that is not working. To perceive the world differently, we must be willing to change our belief system, let the past slip away, expand our sense of now, and dissolve the fear in our minds.* - William James

LOVE and TENDERNESS

Three dozen double blind, randomized studies of couples all demonstrated that when one person focused his loving thoughts and intentions on his partner, the out-of-sight partner's blood flow and perspiration changed within two seconds, as if orienting to a stimulus. The mechanism of action remains unexplained.

> *Love and desire are the spirit's wings to great deeds.* - Johann Wolfgang von Goethe

The chemistry and brain regions involved in feeling love and being loving are those in common with our pleasure centers. Areas such as the anterior insula and anterior cingulate cortex become active both when we feel our own pain and when we know that someone we love is in pain. It involves the dopamine reward system, including the orbital cortex and nucleus accumbens. Whether it be drugs, food, gambling or sex, almost identical reactions occur in the brain, stimulating release of dopamine. Stress evoked hormone CRH and its receptor CRHR1 cause fear in the brain's limbic system, but stimulate the dopamine reward network at same time, creating courage and confidence to counter that fear.

Romantic love, too, is mediated by dopamine and is characterized by craving and focused attention for just one person. And attachment — the bonding and security you feel with a long-term partner — involves neuropetides oxytocin and vasopressin. Oxytocin is the hormone that produces that blissful afterglow following orgasm, and is the same one mothers release when giving birth, and when developing their life-long bond with their baby.

> *Love is metaphysical gravity.* - Buckminster Fuller

Maternal, paternal, familial, divine, societal, spiritual, universal, love — all is our bliss. Compassion, emotional connection, intimacy, empathy — if others will bear witness to our pain, then we are not alone in it. The ultimate sedative, antianxiety, pain reliever, antidepressant, motivator — is love. And this includes the love between an owner and pet. Pets do not care if we are old, incompetent, mentally ill or unattractive. They love us unconditionally.

> *All loves are a bridge to Divine love. Yet, those who have not had a taste of it do not know!* - Jalaluddin Rumi

SPENDING your TIME

And of course, time and attention focused on your patient, dramatically reduces the risk of a malpractice complaint. If there is compassion and human connection, errors and complications can be understood and even forgiven. But lack of acts of humanity — cold objectivity, feeling ignored, rushed and pushed — evokes fear, rage, enmity. It triggers, in your patient, that nasty nocebo response, undermining the effectiveness of you and your treatment.

> Time, Tenderness, Touch … leads to Trust.

BUILDING the SCAFFOLD

The mind's natural state is one of duality. We each tend to see the world with our own preferences, labeling it with extremes of good / bad, right / wrong, love / hate, pain / pleasure, when actually all is just what IS or what eastern philosophies call "suchness." Cognitive dissonance arises from this duality, the holding of two conflicting thoughts in mind — such as rational and irrational — simultaneously. This phenomenon is also called the 'tension of the opposites' and the act of its resolution is called the transcendent function.

THE TRANSCENDENT FUNCTION

In his essay, "The Transcendent Function" Jung described the process of coming to terms with the unconscious as a work that involves both action and suffering. He named it the Transcendent Function because it bridges the gulf between your conscious and your unconscious. It is a natural process, a manifestation of the energy that springs from that tension of the opposites. This process requires a rational mind that can maintain its conviction while in the face of the irrational unconscious. Both are of equal value. We need them both. The confrontation between the two generates an energy, creating a living, third essence. This bringing together of opposites for the production of a third, can be thought of as a dialectic process. The procreation of the species' dependence upon the duality of the sexes, is an illustrious example of the dialectic. The sex act is the transcendent function arising from the duality and the resultant baby is the third essence generated from the 'tension' between them. Got it?

Laura Kragie, MD: Be the Rainbow • Bridge Heaven and Earth

> *There can be no transforming of darkness into light and of apathy into movement without emotion.* - Carl G. Jung

If a person can hold that tension, cognitive dissonance, between the conflicting opposites, then eventually something will happen in the psyche to resolve their conflict. Consistent with our scaffold analogy, we can use the conceptual metaphor of tensengrity, where the creation of the buckyball structure is the resolution of the force vectors. Tension of opposites provides strength and resiliency to the structure, analogous to a bridge. Tensengrity is a great metaphor for the human body too; tension from opposite poles, form rigid infrastructure components. It provides great strength that can withstand deformation. It's not surprising to learn that the new age writer, Carlos Castenada, used this conceptual metaphor to describe the Mexican shamans' integration of physical and spiritual bodies.

> *Don't oppose forces, use them.* - Buckminster Fuller

So how do we actually pull off this transcendent function and resolve these opposites? The trick here is to get your rational mental fovea to BE AWARE of the prevailing conflicting duality. Because you are confident and are assured, you then have control; so tell yourself that you ACCEPT IT, and ALLOW IT TO JUST BE. Then, voilà, no dissonance. Your mind just seems to be cool with it, and goes along with the ride, no longer struggling or resisting each opposite.   EXISTENTIAL SURRENDER happens when you finally, consciously, stop the conflict and with it comes peace, relief, serenity.

Another example to help us understand the dialectic is the wave versus particle duality of light; quantum field theory resolved its paradox. The complementarity principle states that some objects have multiple properties that appear to be contradictory. Sometimes it is possible to switch back and forth between different views of an object to observe these properties, but it is impossible to view both at the same time, despite their simultaneous coexistence in reality. Generally, the fovea-like rational mind does not like the tension and distraction of a paradoxical duality — it wants to focus fully and singly. It generates this tension, cognitive dissonance, and the mind tries to change the input that is coming in to it, to have it coincide with better clarity and coherence.   But note, we CANNOT ASK BOTH QUESTIONS (e.g. wave, particle) AT THE SAME TIME. We need to examine the picture with one perspective first, then the other, then collect both solutions into a synthesis.

> *The battles that count aren't the ones for gold medals. The struggles within yourself — the invisible, inevitable battles inside all of us — that's where it's at.* - Jesse Owens

You actually do this all the time. Think of the concepts of masculinity versus femininity. Be it Mom or Dad, either will instantly go from cuddling their infant (feminine) to fighting off an attack from a wild animal (masculine) threatening that same infant. No problem. You do it without thinking.

> *There are no elements so diverse that they cannot be joined in the heart of a man.* - Jean Giraudoux

Art's Pointillism, as illustrated by works of Seurat, purposely uses complementary (opposite) colors to generate the 'seeing' of the intermediary form (third essence), because it shows more luminosity than when using the intermediary formed from using mixed pigments. You can test this yourself by viewing the two colors juxtaposed, slightly overlapping or very close together. They have the effect of generating another third color when seen from a distance. Note too, that 'halo' that you see after staring at a color, it is actually its opposing, or complementary, color; e.g. you will see the complementary color cyan for a red.

> *Each band or level, being a particular manifestation of the spectrum, is what it is, only by virtue of the other bands. The color blue is no less beautiful because it exists along side the other colors of a rainbow, and "blueness" itself depends upon the existence of the other colors, for if there were no color but blue, we would never be able to see it.* - Ken Wilber

Without opposites, there are no borders to define the entity or idea, all fades into the invisible.

> *It is only with the heart that one can see rightly; what is essential is invisible to the eye.* - Antoine de Saint-Exupery

Figure 1. THE COGNITIVE SCAFFOLD SCHEMATA

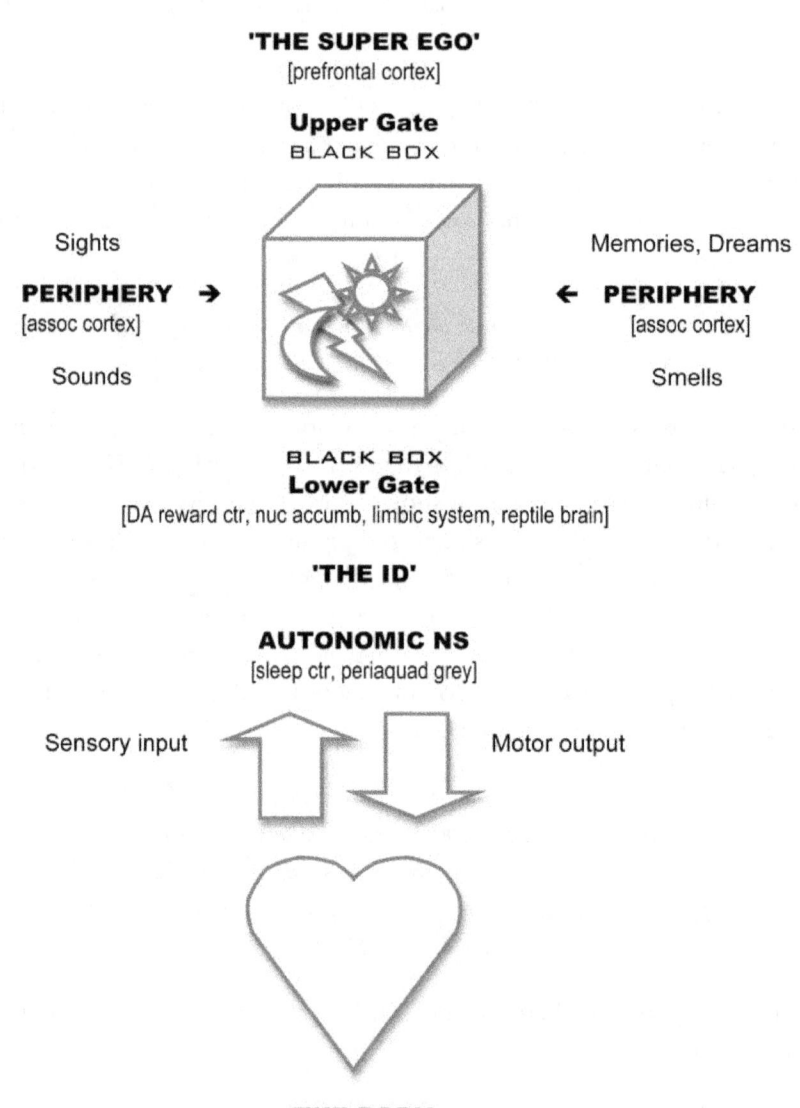

BLACK BOX: YOUR CRUCIBLE

> *Have the courage to take your own thoughts seriously, for they will shape you.* - Albert Einstein

So now, try to visualize a Black Box existing in your mind and that it acts as a machine for your Transcendent Function to generate that third essence arising from the tension of your rational logical fovea-like mind and its peripheral unconscious counterparts. Pilots, soldiers and surgeons are usually trained to compartmentalize their thoughts and emotions, in order to maintain a sharp focus in the face of challenges. But in this case, try a different kind of compartmentalization. Don't make up a secure place to store stuff away; instead actually go INTO that compartment in order to fully experience its contents.

> *Everyone sees the unseen in proportion to the clarity of his heart, and that depends upon how much he has polished it. Whoever has polished it more sees more — more unseen forms become manifest to him.* - Jalaluddin Rumi

So WHAT exactly is in that BLACK BOX?

Your Black Box is a safe place to experience dreams, visions, synesthesias, and moods, without limitation, without analysis and without judgment. To go there, your frontal cortex 'super ego' has to agree to let go and back off control, to allow you the freedom to play in the Box. And it will not do so unless you are not needing its functions at that time. So it's best to choose nap time or meditation time, and not the middle of your presentation to the corporate board or during a heart transplant operation.

> *It's time to lose your mind and come to your senses.* - Fritz Perls

Once in there, you are swimming in your primordial soup of ideas, for you are communing with your 'reptile' brain. Inside your Black Box you can swirl around and marinate in the vast unconscious elements arising from your peripheral mind, those iceberg elements that exist below the rational waterline — giving you access to those contents that your conscious brain cannot usually see. In this space you suspend disbelief, there are no laws of causality, and gravity and other usual rules of reality do not always behave as expected. This pool is the source from which you pull out those potent archetypes, icons, holograms, symbols and metaphors.

Here is where you generate that sense of lift and expansion inside of you when you hear the resounding call of a choir singing Handel's *Messiah* Hallelujah chorus. What occurs is experiential and impressionistic. Here is where the dots of sensation and subliminal memory connect into forms of beliefs, myths, dreams and new creations. Here is where you generate the body sense to hit the homerun or do that funky dance. Here is where all those nonverbal cues and communications turn into your 'gut instinct' making quick judgments.

> *Our normal waking consciousness, rational consciousness as we call it, is but one special type of consciousness, whilst all about it, parted from it by the filmiest of screens, there lie potential forms of consciousness entirely different.* - William James

Your awareness and insight are what allow you to consciously traverse in and out of this Black Box — without them we devolve into delusions and delirium. That is the crucial distinction!

THE GATEWAYS INTO YOUR BLACK BOX

> *There are things known and there are things unknown, and in between are the doors* - Aldous Huxley
> *Be an opener of doors.* - Ralph Waldo Emerson

The whole mind with all its peripheral parts, is really more like a Pointillistic hologram; seeing from multiple perspectives in your mind's eye gives you a 3-D image. You need to develop a holographic view of whatever is your issue or topic in order to see all the facets — just as if it were a crystal. Take for example the many different perspective views of a soldier. The commander sees him as a reliable and efficient weapon, his fellow comrades as a blood brother loyal to the team, his country as an honorable hero, his mother as a young boy vulnerable and mortal, and his enemy as a terrifying monster. He is all these and more, all at once. And, all these perspectives co-exist in the mind's eye of that same soldier.

To access those many perspectives, you need to communicate with your Black Box contents — pull back the veil. And that veil is not over the view of the outer world, but instead, over each of our eyes — the veil being

Laura Kragie, MD: Be the Rainbow • Bridge Heaven and Earth

actually our own minds. By becoming aware of the Box and its gates, we clear away that obscuring web.

> *When the doors of perception are cleansed, Man will see things as they truly are, infinite.* - William Blake

UPPER GATE

Visualize the entrance to your sanctum. Pull back the curtain and enter the soothing dark hallway. To get into your Black Box and create your novel solution, take a hot shower, meander, daydream, stare out at nature's beauty, go running, work your garden, follow the idle moves of fish — whatever it takes to damp down your frontal cortices running those oh-so-important executive functions. Enter that stage of twilight between wakefulness and sleep.

> *I think present-day reason is an analogue of the flat earth of the medieval period. If you go too far beyond it you're presumed to fall off, into insanity.* - Robert M. Pirsig

Because you are mindful, YOU HAVE COMPLETE CONTROL as to when and whether you enter and leave your box. Remember that it's your awareness and your insight that distinguishes this 'exercise' from insanity, psychosis, and drugged states. Think of this as being similar to Lucid Dreaming, like in the movie, Inception. The fovea of your mind, is the super surveillant, super consciousness. That rational mind kept the cave man alive back when we were all living on the Serengeti. It will keep track of your mind's meandering and bring you safely back to focus and clarity, at your discretion and direction.

LOWER GATE

> *Action seems to follow feeling, but really action and feeling go together; and by regulating the action, which is under the more direct control of the will, we can indirectly regulate the feeling, which is not.* - William James

In your Black Box you also have a conduit to its Lower Gate — access to the old reptile brain (that includes your the medial forebrain pleasure circuit) and autonomic nervous system. It is the venue and route for that Embodiment phenomena to pervade our thoughts and language. And this lower gate is consciously and deliberately accessible to experienced yogi gurus, achieved over a lifetime of training.

Yoga Nidra promotes awareness during the process of sleeping, including those stages of deep sleep. Its practice lengthens your time spent in the stages between wakefulness and sleep. It encourages you to examine your thought patterns, control your breath, and generate proprioceptive awareness throughout your body, in the absence of external stimuli. Yoga gurus, have succeeded in consciously producing delta waves thus demonstrating that they can deliberately alter their own brain state, while remaining fully conscious during stages that are characteristic of a deep sleep state. And with Hatha Yoga practices your ideal is to gain nearly complete control over the body's every function. Incredible control over autonomic nervous system and nonstriated muscles is possible.

It seems as if these extreme states are a form of human hibernation, characterized by increases in the parasympathetic, and decreases in the sympathetic, systems. Going along with this is a bump in GABA, consistent with the physiologic changes seen with the Relaxation Response. These yogis can reduce the amounts of their exhaled CO_2 from the normal 4% down to 2%. Yogic practice leads to enhanced parasympathetic activities, stabilizes autonomic balance during stress, and improves thermoregulation efficiency. You can see the therapeutic potential of these yogic practices for the control and management of, e.g. hypertension.

> *If the grace of God miraculously operates, it probably operates through the subliminal door.* - William James

The Stravinsky acting method touches on those sense memories embodied in the physical body that are triggered by sensory stimuli. Similarly, ambient conditions and activated senses can trigger a cascade of 'gut feelings' that feed into our judgment calls, without even our conscious awareness. For example, we will be 'soft' on an employee if we are sitting in a comfortable chair or rate a new hire as warm and friendly, if we are holding a warm cup of tea. Such is the power of the body's feedback coming through the lower gate, into that sloppy soup of the Black Box.

GARDEN of EDEN LESSONS

When we took that bite of apple from the Tree of Knowledge, we left Paradise (our Black Box!) to live in the rational state or 'earth world' — hence, losing our innocence, and gaining the negativity surrounding all such worldly knowledge. We need to know that we can return, for a time, to that place of wonder. It is not gone, entirely.

Just remember when you are in each world, you do have to strap on a different toolbelt, a different mindset, one apropos to the question and to the milieu. KNOWING when you are in each 'world' is the AWARENESS, your INSIGHT. Sanity absolutely requires this awareness, for without it, we are then plunged instead into a state of delirium, delusion or confusion.

Metaphorically, the Black Box requires housekeeping, i.e. mental hygiene — especially for dealing with any 'flooding up from the sewer, through the lower gate.' Be vigilant and patrol the neighborhood of your Black Box, keeping out the vermin and dis-ease. Use your heaven tools like yoga, meditation, prayer, play, and love to fill your Black Box with sunshine and clean air, so it will sprout bright healthy ideas and creations.

Luck favors the prepared mind. - Louis Pasteur

Scientists often express that they were lucky, because so many scientific discoveries are stumbled upon, rather than sought out. From your experience and observation while in your Black Box, you can then return back to your fovea-like rational mind, but now more enriched with the gift of your creativity. Connect your Black Box inner thoughts with your rational conscious mind so that you can communicate to others what you have found. Like the rainbow, the riches come from what it creates as it links heaven and earth (the third essence) and not any pot of gold at its nonexistent end. Your rewards arise from your Black Box efforts.

Imagination is more important than knowledge, for while knowledge defines everything we know and understand, imagination points to all we might yet discover and create. - Albert Einstein

BASIC HOW-TO'S: RAINBOW PRACTITIONER™ LOGISTICS

Clear eyes, full heart, can't lose. - Friday Night Lights

OK now, back to earth. Pragmatics. Time for putting it all together, into your everyday practice. Let's start with the players.

THE RAINBOW PRACTITIONER™

You are now a Healer who wants to navigate between and within the two worlds to best serve your clients' needs. You have mentally constructed a cognitive scaffold, allowing you to peacefully integrate 'Heaven and Earth' and allow the simultaneous benefit of both. You have achieved that ultimate 'aha! moment' when you transcended the paradoxical duality of rational-irrational thought, allowing them to coexist peacefully.

Paradox = Pair of Docs ;-)

Your success is operationally defined. And you don't bother to 'wax philosophically' about the 'mechanism of action' of the beneficial synergy provided by belief. You just apply the knowledge we have gained to-date, and let it help to relieve the suffering of the world. Your goals are phenomenalistic. So as you apply the tools, evaluate your outcomes: Did your resource management and allocations change? Are you are more willing to collaborate with a nonmedical healer in order to help a client? Have you found trusted alternative health practitioners more able and willing to affiliate with your standard medical setting? Are there fewer

Laura Kragie, MD: Be the Rainbow • Bridge Heaven and Earth

adverse events and therapeutic failures? Fewer disgruntled patients and complaints?

THE RAINBOW PRACTICE TEAM MEMBERS

> *I will make company with creators, with harvesters, with rejoicers; I will show them the rainbow and the stairway to the Superman.* - Friedrich Nietzsche

Who is your Client/Patient? This is someone who seeks a holistic therapeutic approach to their personal wellness; takes on some of the responsibility for their own health; and works collaboratively with your team to build trust and belief in a good outcome.

Who are your Healthcare Colleagues? Your Earth Workers or Medical Docs (MDs) —collectively, 'Mainstream Medicine' — are scientists, doctors, and health professionals trained in evidence-based medicine, rooted to the rational scientific approaches to relieve disease and suffering, who may not yet be oriented to incorporate 'nonrational' therapeutics into their practices.

Who are your Heaven Helpers (HHs)? These are the Spiritual Practitioners seeking an understanding of, and reconciliation with, mainstream medicine; healers whose therapeutic practices and efficacy are based on belief in a higher power and/or facilitates the client's self healing using their inner resources. What are they NOT? They are NOT lay folks pretending to be licensed medical doctors! As well, HHs are NOT psychics, gods, goddesses, oracles, gurus, superhumans, saints, or miracle workers.

Here are some hypothetical HHs to consider for your Rainbow Practice Team:

- Moms, to kiss away the booboo's, to soothe and to cradle the babies.

- That phenomenal and popular nurse who is way out there on the touchy-feely spectrum.

- The Zen meditating monk, who can effectively calm and teach your patient, using breath and body techniques.

Laura Kragie, MD: Be the Rainbow • Bridge Heaven and Earth

- Therapeutic massage / physical therapists with all-knowing and magic hands, who can think out-of-box and customize an approach to heal your patient's problems and pain.

- Acupuncturists, attuned to the power of the needle in affecting the mind of those patients open to this path.

- Spiritual counselors, shamans and priests of all varieties and faiths that take a positive, loving approach to healing.

- Health coaches, social workers and teams to provide social support and to tap into the energy of the mob.

- Movement Makers of all kinds: dancers, yoga instructors, martial artists, sports teams, your playful dog.

- Online games and communities, including: WoW, Words with Friends, Sim World, especially for shut-ins and the bedridden.

- Music therapists of all kinds: to help the aphasics, to provide social bonding in chorus, to help gait training in rehab, to trance with twirls or drums, to treat moods, for comfort and for pleasure.

- Art therapists, occupational therapists and kinesiologists who can think 'out of the box' when needed.

- Higher Power 12 step programs for all addictions, harnessing the good from groups and gods.

- Divination artists who help develop subliminal skills such as lucid dreaming, journaling, artwork, tarot cards, I Ching, and runes.

- Smart phone apps: e.g. for health coaching, prayer for the day/affirmations, breathing meditations, yoga, journaling, art, gaming, binaural beats.

- Animal Therapists, including horses, puppies, kittens, parrots, canaries and all those creatures found in the beauty of the great outdoors or your own Garden of Eden (hummingbirds, butterflies...).

Laura Kragie, MD: Be the Rainbow • Bridge Heaven and Earth

> *Dogs are our link to paradise. They don't know evil or jealousy or discontent. To sit with a dog on a hillside on a glorious afternoon is to be back in Eden, where doing nothing was not boring — it was peace.* - Milan Kundera

THE RAINBOW PRACTICE - TEAM ROLES DEFINED

For the sake of clarity and understanding, we compare and contrast these hypothetical roles and personas of your Earth Workers (MDs) and your Heaven Helpers (HHs). There are sharply defined distinctions. Clearly, when functioning as a Medical Doctor there are LOTS of regulatory constraints, regulations, certifications, audits, and oversight imposed on the medical practice. Some of these include:

- Hippocratic oath swears MDs to a set of ethics.

- A doctor-patient relationship is implied with each encounter, and hence all fall under those applicable laws and liabilities.

- HIPAA regulates and constrains how health information and patient privacy must be protected.

- The 1986 Emergency Medical Treatment and Active Labor Act (EMTALA) demands that MDs practicing at hospitals must treat all patients in need, despite any inability to pay.

- Standards of the medical practice are as dictated from the Tort Court; MDs can be sued if they do not practice similarly to other MDs.

- Medical License regulations require continuous medical education, having no significant disabilities, and having no criminal record.

- Speciality Boards require regular retesting and recertification.

- Federal agencies AQPR and CMS dictate practice guidelines and what will be reimbursed and for how much.

- Federal agency FDA restricts labeling and the use of approved medicines and devices.

Laura Kragie, MD: Be the Rainbow • Bridge Heaven and Earth

- Managed Care organizations dictate the time allotted per patient and extent of care.

- Payment diagnostic codes construct and direct the doctor-patient encounter.

- Malpractice and litigation threats push the need to practice defensive medicine and over-testing.

Now, in stark contrast, when one is functioning as a Heaven Helper using the faith-based healing modalities, there are very few constraints, obligations or responsibilities:

- There are no official academic or professional degrees to obtain to become a HH.

- There is no legal oversight dictating your HH practice.

- There is no legal obligation to provide free care to those who cannot / will not pay.

- HHs and their teachers use the feedback obtained from many years of practice to assess the quality of their techniques, and not the government agencies or legal courts.

- HHs do not need to focus on mechanisms of action or scientific cause and effect and instead, concentrate on a phenomenalistic and individualistic approach to the client.

- HH techniques are heavily based on 'faith' — i.e. NOT on scientifically testable hypotheses.

- HH clients require the use of their Black Box and heaven toolset in order to manifest the HH's treatment 'efficacy' – i.e. how they feel, their emotive and cognitive states, their depth of relaxation.

So then, how should we evaluate each type of practice? How should we dispense each? Medical docs are constrained by tort law, the cost of medical malpractice insurance and standard of care practices; they must document everything for reimbursement (if MDs use the wrong codes, they can be arrested). BUT this is not the case for the Heaven Helper (HH).

They are free to practice however and whenever they choose. Therefore, HHs really need to understand the constraints, conduct and quality of practice that is required to work collaboratively with MDs in their setting and their situation. HHs need to be aware and supportive of the regulations and ethics associated with patient healthcare. However, HHs truly are at their best when they can fill in those gaps created by all these restrictions and obstacles placed upon the standard medical practice. HHs working flexibly with MDs can really enhance the team's quality, and their ability to reach goals and to reduce costs effectively. But this will not occur unless HHs learn, understand and empathize with the MDs' professional constraints and obligations.

As a Rainbow Practitioner™ your CMS reimbursement will be tied to quality outcome measures under the ACA. You will have to measure them anyway, so use these data to assess your own approaches to and techniques for the individual patient — what works for them? Use these data to give them, and your team, essential feedback. Seek to find the common component that leads to the most potent effects. Sort through the informatics to search for outcome measures and use them to compare the presence and absence of the HH contributions. The combination of HH with MD also allows for the 'good cop, bad cop routine,' which can be very useful at times, especially dealing with addictions.

BUT underpinning the foundations and applications of this powerful Heaven toolset is the Ethical Credo for all the team members: Duty to Distinguish and Disclose.

ETHICAL CREDO: DISCERN and DISCLOSE

I see your true colors shining through. Don't be afraid, let them show, your True Colors. True Colors, are beautiful, like a rainbow. - Cyndi Lauper

Use of both these 'toolsets' are linked to an overarching Ethical Credo that pledges to Distinguish and Disclose the basis of the particular therapeutic approach that the Rainbow Practitioner™ chooses to use with each therapeutic encounter. Here, the emphasis must be on transparency of action and intent, and the ethical communication of these, to your client. Be transparent — about your basis for recommendation, your role, your approach. This Credo is applied here, in addition to all the usual standards of practice. Patient centered care, shared decision-making, outcome-based billing — all these will help to establish trust between healer and healed.

The Rainbow Practitioner™ will often face the pragmatic problem of whether to disclose to their client, the concept and likelihood of placebo effects. If needed, you may say honestly, that you do not personally believe, but that you can accept other's beliefs. You can allow to occur, any positive synergy of Heaven Helper actions, when they are performed in collaboration with standard evidence-based medicine. Again remember, therapeutic outcome is based on that individual patient's response (RCT statistics are based on the population's response) and is phenomenalistic regarding that particular individual. So, Disclose your take on things. If you are not supportive of your patient's beliefs, they will hide them from you, and work against your recommendations, perhaps even to prove you wrong and their beliefs right. Yes, do inform your patients about the nocebo effect (or call it by its other name, Medical Student Syndrome) just as you would the more positive placebo effect. Let your patient use their beliefs, but coach them with PMA to use their 'Spidey Powers' for good.

Respect your patient's views enough to allow a Heaven Helper teammate to coordinate with your patient to have their beliefs function as an adjunct to the prescribed mainstream medical therapy. And you Heaven Helpers, please be happy to be who you are. Be proud to practice your own thing, and please don't pretend to be what you are not. Be trustworthy, to your teammates, to your client / patient. *Primum non nocere*. Of course, **First Do No Harm**!

Be self-aware and be conscious of where you are coming from. Let your 'True Colors' show through. You MUST honestly Distinguish and Disclose the distinctly different personas — MD vs. HH — when dispensing medicine, therapy or advice. Otherwise you are being dishonest, for you know each approach is evaluated very differently.

But, when asked how it all works, remember that "I don't know" is an okay answer!

> *I wish there were a way to make "I don't know" a positive thing, which it isn't in our society. We feel that we need to "know" certain things, and we substitute that quest for the actual experience of things in all its complexity.*

Laura Kragie, MD: Be the Rainbow • Bridge Heaven and Earth

> *When I play pure improvisation, any kind of intellectual handles are inappropriate because they get in the way of letting the river move where it's supposed to move.* - Keith Jarrett, jazz artist

Using your best overall clinical judgment that is pertinent to the individual, is okay too. In fact, it is more than okay, because your judgment now includes all that creativity and gut instinct gained from diving into your own Black Box.

> *Be patient toward everything unresolved in your heart and try to love the questions themselves. Do not search for the answers which could not be given to you now because you would not be able to live them. And the point is to live everything ... Live the questions now. Perhaps you will then gradually, without noticing it, evolve some distant day into the answer.* - Rainer Maria Rilke

RAINBOW PRACTITIONER™ EXAMPLE SCENARIOS

So bottom-line, it's time to 'get back to the future.' Seems it's 'deja vu all over again', where 'everything old is new again.' Remember Bush Senior's Thousand Points of Light? We need to get back to having lots of good, competent, caring nurses; bring back the dedicated nuns, candy stripers, the parish, church and temple involvement. Bring back extended family members supporting the care of their sick ones. Exploit that heaven toolset!

> *If you want to teach people a new way of thinking, don't bother trying to teach them. Instead, give them a tool, the use of which will lead to new ways of thinking.* - Buckminster Fuller

Here are some fictional scenarios to help you get started in brainstorming some new ways to enhance your own practice.

Sedona Red Canyons Vortex of Vibration. Mark didn't really know why he came here. The job he left was good money. And his wife ... well, he just didn't want to be there, anymore. What was the purpose of the work, the struggle? Where did his passion for life, go? "Here at the Vortex, we'll explore the recesses of your amazing minds. You can enhance your lucid dreaming output with some work at the Tarot cards, I Ching or Celtic

Runes. Tomorrow, our shamans have scheduled an overnight hike into the canyons where, hopefully, you'll commune with the spirit of Carlos Castenadas, and contemplate his message, "For me the world is weird because it is stupendous, awesome, mysterious, unfathomable; my interest has been to convince you that you must assume responsibility for being here, in this marvelous world, in this marvelous desert, in this marvelous time. I want to convince you that you must learn to make every act count, since you are going to be here for only a short while, in fact, too short for witnessing all the marvels of it."

Airport Disaster Command Center after an Emergency Landing. The place was filling up now with the passengers streaming in after just being bussed in from the landing site. Their eyes went wide as soon as they turned the corner. There was a pen filled with bunnies and chicks! It had been set up temporarily there for an Easter-themed petting zoo. None of them could pass by the furry balls without picking up one to pet and cuddle. I looked at the medic, "Why aren't you taking their vitals?" "No way. I know their BPs are sky high. Just give 'em all a bit of time with the babies; trust me, it will really cut down on any needed trips to the ER."

Journaling Class - Writing to Save your Life. "When we're faced with a really traumatic memory it gets pushed aside because your mind doesn't know how to deal with it. But, if you access that memory using creativity, you can distance yourself from the painful parts. You can take your story and shape it into a better way. Re-See it and write a different, less nightmarish ending." Karen was dealing with memories of the car crash. She was on an icy hill, heading down towards the river, when it crashed through the guardrail, the water bubbled up to her windows ... "In the story, as I write it this time, I am rescued by the police before the water seeps into the car. Before I nearly drown." "Is it working for you?" "Yes. I am beginning to feel, now, like the movie director, instead of the actor in the nightmare. I have some control."

Yes We Can, Kick Addiction Rehab Center. Whether it be drugs, food, gambling or sex, almost identical reactions occur in the brain. So here, in this residence nestled in the serene beauty of the Big Sur, we replace 'em with a healthier set of dopamine pumpers. While doing your detox and withdrawal, you can seek out your Higher Power 24/7 with any of our 12

Laura Kragie, MD: Be the Rainbow • Bridge Heaven and Earth

Steppers, Zen Meditation, Quigong, Taiji, and yoga classes. The Outward Bound rock climbing, hikes, team sports, and martial art workouts continuously challenge you to stay sober. "And may the odds be EVER in your favor."

Post-Partum Life. The sun's rays cut through the drapes, stabbing Mom in her tired, barely closed eyes. The colicky toddler could be heard crying in the background. Ding-dong, Mom opens the front door and sighs with relief. "Hey Girlfriend. Saw your tweet and figured you could use reinforcements to help get you and baby Chuck through teething. I brought along Mikey." The two BFFs sit down to sip one more mug of caffeine, while the two toddlers migrate towards the TV.   On comes Beyonce ... and lo and behold ... the boys are wildly bouncing along, giggling to *All the Single Ladies*. Mom smiles, and those tired lines begin to ease from her face.

The Body Consultant. Irina the Ballerina was hard at work with her Alexander Technique consulting practice. She glanced over her gathering of clients, all computer geeks hunched over their smart phones like pretzels, in pain. "Soon, you will see, I will transform you. You will lightly elevate from your chairs like heavenly angels and glide smoothly across the floor, as if on skates. Pain and stiffness will ease away."

Bethesda Medical Center. The door to the Walter Reed PT gym was open and out blared Lady Gaga's *Telephone*. Glancing in, it's hard to tell who is the patient and who the therapist — looks more like a dance party is going on. The kinesiologists had linked up with some local dancers to help with the gait training. And one vet was really getting into it, "Those new prosthetics sure are bouncy, just like a rubber band, helps me keep up my rhythm, my swag. Never miss a beat!"

The Independent Charter School. "For these autistics' schooling, we brought in actual teachers of Method Acting for we are, essentially, all method actors who understand others by simulating the responses we see in them. People in conversations begin to mimic the body language of the other person, and the more closely they mimic the other's body language, the more perceptive they are about the other person's emotions. For the stutterers, we have rappers coming in tomorrow to volunteer some of their time."

Laura Kragie, MD: Be the Rainbow • Bridge Heaven and Earth

Geriatric Play Land. Folks from the assisted living center strolled across the grounds to the co-located Kids Daycare facility. The playground soon got populated with smiling seniors spotting for the rambunctious little ones, who were spinning madly around the merry-go-round. They stumbled off giggling, still twirling and dizzy, and nipping at their heels to herd the stray ones away from the boundaries, was their beloved mascot, a Sheltie dog.

Posted at the front desk of the University Mental Health Clinic: "Our staff includes a canine therapist. He is without vanity and ambition, has no 'pet' theories, is unconcerned with role or status, is free of intellectual pretensions, does not fear emotion and does not feel that he is being underpaid."

Dr. Pain Reliever Clinic and Spa. "Bring us your aches and pains; you'll leave them behind when you go. We have saunas to bake out your stiffness and hot tubs to steep out the toxins. And our therapists have just the right massage for your muscles. In between, there is stretching and restorative yoga sessions, nature walks during the day and dance parties at night. We'll renew you."

Move That Groove, Weight Loss Cooperative. Mavis the manager, herded up her new pack of the depressed obese and headed them out to the dance floor. She was determined to turn them around this time. "Alright, I wanna hear ya loud clear, repeat after me, 'shake that booty'..." and so it went in her Jazzercize session. She closed the class dancing to Amy Grant's *Every Heartbeat Belongs to You*. "And now perhaps you'll actually have many more."

Cat in the Hat Pediatric Urgent Care Center. The aquarium quietly bubbles, as the angelfish idle by. In her lap, Mom is comforting and cosseting her toddler Tessa, who is laying her head on Mom's breast, listening and feeling her humming *Amazing Grace*. Doc stealthily, quickly, efficiently reaches over and sets the baby's greenstick wrist fracture.

Your Community Horse Stable. These Wounded Warriors love caring for and riding their horses. They breathe in all the nature and enjoy hearing the birds sing. Their outreach extends to supporting their community by volunteering to ride the caissons at funerals for veterans. "I feel like I am back in time, when we had a cavalry in the military. When riding, I am one with my war horse; I totally forget that I don't have my leg."

Pediatric Intensive Care Unit. The mother was sobbing at her baby's bedside, the cries now reaching that hysterical pitch, with hiccupping. Sister Mary Elizabeth shook her head and wondered, who was it that left her alone there? Quietly, she placed her arm around the bent shoulders. "Let me sit with you. The antibiotics are now running through your child, battling that meningitis. For now, all we can do is let go and let God. Let's pray the rosary together.

THE TAKE AWAYS

You may want to find a good HH and emulate their bedside manner; personally, I learned a lot during my own teenage years spent waitressing. But maybe you are more the Vulcan Science Officer Spock, than the Baby Doc Spock. It's okay. Be true to your nature, because it may be that this is what allows you to be so good in the OR and ER. Just be sure to include on your Rainbow team, those who may have what you lack — such as those who have the capacity to withstand intense waves of tough emotions like grief and pain. No school can grant a certificate or degree signifying this ability, because there is no course to 'teach' and 'test' for it. But the comfort provided to your patient is priceless.

Apply your tools appropriately and efficiently; square peg in round hole just won't work. When should we use each? The example from **Zen and Art of Motorcycle Maintenance** teaches us that it is futile to try to rationalize and define beauty or art or quality of rhetoric. Just recognize it. DO use rational, scientific tools to explore specific structured questions and testable hypotheses, where you can isolate and control variables of interest, and measure all pertinent outcomes. For example, setup a drug allergy / side effect protocol for an individual patient. Record effects and timeline, then carefully watch as you reintroduce each suspect agent to suss out the offender. Use your individual clinical expertise — the proficiency and judgment that you as a clinician acquired through your years of training and practice. And when choosing therapies, remember that generic and nonpatented products are in the public domain, but are usually NOT studied because there is no profit to be made. So be aware that these other therapies are out there to use, only we cannot rely on having lots of great gold standard data to use in evaluating them.

> *The important thing is not to stop questioning. Curiosity has its own reason for existing.* - Albert Einstein

As a Rainbow Practitioner™, you will need to balance out the use of your earth and heaven tools when deciding how best to guide your patient. Do not lose that window of opportunity for the gain resulting from using the earth tools, when you delay treatment to try heaven tools, e.g. in treating cancer. But also, do not let unnecessary adverse reactions occur from using earth products (e.g. drugs) when the illness could have been better dealt with using heaven tools (e.g. for depression). Disclose all the reasonable risks you know, and these include the risks of not using the earth tools in time and where appropriate. Remind your patient that organic substances and high doses of supplements are STILL drugs and not heaven tools; they must be interpreted as being more earth tools, especially if they disrupt normal healthy homeostasis.

So what to do? Be open-minded, and be skeptical, even of the established dogma. Use your heaven tools and your time in the Black Box to come up with new ideas. Use your earth tools to test out your hypotheses of what will most likely work for your individual patient. Then evaluate the outcomes, and learn.

> *Everyone knows that on any given day there are energies slumbering in him which the incitements of that day do not call forth. Compared with what we ought to be, we are only half awake. The human individual usually lives far within his limits.* - William James

Find creative solutions when the gold standards and established procedures are just not available to you. Consider this example, pulled from experience at a small pharma company where we were tasked to very quickly assemble all the patient safety data from an ongoing clinical trial for submission to the FDA. All the data existed on paper in storage warehouses. It was impossible! But then ... we remembered that old infamous aphorism of Willie Sutton, 'go where the money is'. It suddenly dawned on us that the diagnostic testing company knew all our missing data — they had put it into an electronic spreadsheet and sent it to us each week to justify their billing.

Laura Kragie, MD: Be the Rainbow • Bridge Heaven and Earth

So, by pulling up their electronic billing data files from our clinical subjects' blood draw visits, we very quickly and easily created an database of all the trial subjects and their visit dates. The result was nearly perfect in accuracy!

Don't be afraid to use those heaven tools; we do need all the help we can get, for our patients ... and for ourselves. Most of all, be hopeful!

> *Hope is not prognostication. It is an orientation of the spirit, and orientation of the heart; it transcends the world that is immediately experienced, and is anchored somewhere beyond its horizons.* -Vaclav Havel

Rainbow Practioner Tips:

Be Transparent

Be a Team

Build Trust

Benefit from Tolerance

NOT either / or, but INTEGRATE into being the bridge, a Rainbow Practitioner™, using

Time, Tenderness, Touch

NOW to LEARN MORE ... SCIENTIFIC and CULTURAL TIDBITS

This manual is a just a small hint at what is available. So much more is in the literature and media. Here I list resources dense with information and authority, but still entertaining.

The Mother Lode! NPR's *RadioLab* and *On Being/Speaking of Faith*

NPR's *RadioLab*: PODCASTS are at:
http://www.radiolab.org/series/podcasts/ and also iTunes store.

"*Radiolab* believes your ears are a portal to another world. Where sound illuminates ideas, and the boundaries blur between science, philosophy, and human experience. Big questions are investigated, tinkered with, and encouraged to grow. Bring your curiosity, and we'll feed it with possibility." Hosted by NPR Science Correspondent, Robert Krulwich and Jad Abumrad Abumrad (Macarthur genius fellow).

http://www.radiolab.org/2007/may/17/ *Placebo.* From the symbolic power of the doctor coat, to the very real stash of opium in your brain, this hour of Radiolab explores the healing powers of belief and imagination.

http://www.radiolab.org/2007/may/07/ *Who Am I?* The "mind" and "self" were formerly the domain of philosophers and priests. But in this hour of Radiolab, neurologists lead the charge. We reflect on the illusion of selfhood, contemplate the evolution of consciousness, and meet a woman who one day woke up as a completely different person.

Laura Kragie, MD: Be the Rainbow • Bridge Heaven and Earth

http://www.radiolab.org/2006/may/05/ *Where Am I?* Under high gravity forces, fighter pilots often lose consciousness while flying jet planes. Radiolab, examines the connection between your brain and your body...and what happens when it breaks.

http://www.radiolab.org/2011/apr/18/ *Desperately Seeking Symmetry.* Jad and Robert set out in search of order and balance in the world around us, and ask how symmetry shapes our very existence — from the origins of the universe, to what we see when we look in the mirror.

http://www.radiolab.org/2011/mar/08/ *Help!* What do you do when your own worst enemy is ... you? Radiolab looks for ways to gain the upper hand over those forces inside us — from unhealthy urges, to creative insights — that seem to have a mind of their own.

http://www.radiolab.org/2007/may/24/ *Sleep.* Sleep is one of science's greatest mysteries. This hour of Radiolab, we look for answers in iguanas who doze with one eye open, new parents in the throes of sleep deprivation, and rats who may be dreaming.

http://www.radiolab.org/blogs/radiolab-blog/2012/jan/23/wake-up-dream/ *Wake Up and Dream.* Steve Volk was reading through old sleep studies conducted by a scientist named Stephen LaBerge, and he was starting to wonder if lucid dreaming might not be so fringe-y after all.

http://www.radiolab.org/2007/apr/09/ *Stress.* Stress may save your life if you're being chased by a tiger. But if you're stuck in traffic, it may be more likely to make you sick. This hour of Radiolab, stories of stress — from a singer who loses her voice, to an author caught in a body that never grew up.

http://www.radiolab.org/2007/sep/24/sound-as-touch/ *Sound As Touch.* We at Radiolab did our own study of infant-directed speech, recording more than a dozen different parents. The melodies of these recordings illustrate Fernald's findings that there are a set of common tunes living within the words that parents all over the world intone to their babies.

http://www.radiolab.org/2007/sep/24/ *Musical Language.* Radiolab: we explore the line between music and language, and turn to physics and biochemistry to ask how sound becomes feeling.

Laura Kragie, MD: Be the Rainbow • Bridge Heaven and Earth

http://www.radiolab.org/blogs/radiolab-blog/2011/jul/26/4-track-mind/ *A 4-Track Mind.* A neurologist issues a dare to a ragtime piano player and a famous conductor. When the two men face off in an fMRI machine, the challenge is so unimaginably difficult that one man instantly gives up. But the other achieves a musical feat that ought to be impossible.

http://www.radiolab.org/blogs/radiolab-blog/2010/sep/07/voices-in-your-head/ *Voices in Your Head.* Jad talks to Charles Fernyhough about the connection between thought and the voice in your head. How did it get there? And what's happening when people hear someone else's voice in their head?

http://www.radiolab.org/2010/aug/09/ *Words.* It's almost impossible to imagine a world without words. But in this hour of Radiolab, we try to do just that. A woman teaches a 27-year-old the first words of his life, and a neurologist suffers a stroke that wipes out the language center of her brain.

http://www.radiolab.org/blogs/radiolab-blog/2010/may/05/vanishing-words/ *Vanishing Words.* When scientists treat words like data, clues to the real-life mysteries of human aging are found in the writings of Agatha Christie and 678 nuns.

http://www.radiolab.org/blogs/radiolab-blog/2010/mar/08/do-i-know-you/ *Do I Know You?* A rare and haunting disorder called Capgras turns loved ones into imposters — and reveals that recognizing people, even the people we know the best, is more about how they make us feel than what we see in front of our eyes.

http://www.radiolab.org/blogs/radiolab-blog/2010/jun/15/strangers-in-the-mirror/ *Strangers in the Mirror.* Oliver Sacks, the famous neuroscientist and author, can't recognize faces. Neither can Chuck Close — the great artist known for his enormous paintings of ... that's right, faces.

http://www.radiolab.org/2007/jun/07/ *Memory and Forgetting.* Remembering is a tricky, unstable business. This hour of Radiolab: implanting false memories in loved ones, and erasing painful memories by simply swallowing a pill. Plus: the story of a man with the worst case of amnesia ever documented.

http://www.radiolab.org/2008/feb/25/ *Laughter.* Radiolab teases out stories of laughter — from a baby's crib, to a rat's cage, to a remote village in Tanzania that was struck by a laughing epidemic 45 years ago.

http://www.radiolab.org/2008/nov/17/ *Choice*. When presented with a choice, logic and emotion pipe up. This hour of Radiolab, we turn up the volume on those voices in our heads, and try to get to the bottom of what really steers our decisions.

http://www.radiolab.org/blogs/radiolab-blog/2011/jan/11/universe-knows-my-name/ *The Universe Knows My Name*. In this new short, we explore luck and fate, both good and bad, with an author and a cartoon character.

http://www.radiolab.org/2009/jun/15/ *Stochasticity*. Stochasticity is a wonderfully slippery and smarty-pants word for randomness. This hour of Radiolab: making sense of the patterns we see — from lucky streaks to gambling odds, to two girls named Laura.

http://www.radiolab.org/2011/may/31/ *Talking to Machines*. What can machines tell us about being human? This hour of Radiolab, Jad and Robert meet humans and robots who are trying to connect, and blur the line.

http://www.radiolab.org/blogs/radiolab-blog/2010/jul/26/secrets-of-success/ *Secrets of Success*. Robert and Malcolm Gladwell duke it out over questions of luck, talent, passion, and success.

http://www.radiolab.org/2008/dec/29/ *Diagnosis*. In this day and age, we have astonishing technology — chemicals and computers and machines that can pinpoint things imperceptible to our senses. But humans aren't obsolete — intuition and creativity still lead the way both in discovering the nature of the problem, and in dealing with that knowledge.

NPR's ON BEING / SPEAKING OF FAITH PROGRAMS

On Being is a spacious conversation — and an evolving media space — about the big questions at the center of human life, from the boldest new science of the human brain to the most ancient traditions of the human spirit. What does it mean to be human? What matters in a life? What matters in a death? How to love? How to be of service to each other and to the world? The program began in 1999, and launched as a weekly program titled *Speaking of Faith* in the summer of 2003.

FOR PODCASTS: at http://being.publicradio.org and also iTunes store

Investigating Healthy Minds with Richard Davidson (June 23, 2011)
Neuroscientist Richard Davidson explores how the mind can be rewired by life-enriching behaviors.

The Biology of the Spirit (January 18, 2007) Sherwin Nuland on the spirit as an evolutionary accomplishment of the brain.

Einstein's God (December 5, 2005) Freeman Dyson and Paul Davies explore Einstein's way of thinking about mystery, eternity, and the mind of God.

Mathematics, Purpose, and Truth (January 10, 2008) Janna Levin on Godel, Turing, and the paradox of truth.

The Heart's Reason: Hinduism and Science (November 22, 2007) V. V. Raman on Hinduism and science.

Quarks and Creation (April 20, 2006) Physicist John Polkinghorne on modern physics and prayer.

Approaching Prayer (May 22, 2008) Anoushka Shankar, Stephen Mitchell, and Roberta Bondi open up the subject of prayer.

Heart and Soul: The Integrative Medicine of Dr. Mehmet Oz (June 22, 2006) Mehmet Oz on Western medicine, spirituality, and the human heart.

Heart and Soul: The Integrative Medicine of Dr. Mehmet Oz (August 30, 2007) Mehmet Oz looks to traditions and technologies to advance modern medicine.

Stress and the Balance Within (January 12, 2006) Esther Sternberg discusses new scientific insight into the molecular level of the mind-body connection.

The Spirituality of Addiction and Recovery (July 27, 2006) Basil Brave Heart on indigenous spiritual practices and recovery and Susan Cheever on Bill W.

Laura Kragie, MD: Be the Rainbow • Bridge Heaven and Earth

The Spirituality of Addiction and Recovery (May 15, 2008) Buddhist teacher Kevin Griffin on the consonance of the Twelve Steps and Zen instruction; and Susan Cheever tells her personal story and that of her father, the late fiction writer John Cheever.

Play, Spirit, and Character (August 23, 2007) Stuart Brown on the importance of play.

Learning, Doing, Being - A New Science of Education (November 19, 2009) Neuroscientist Adele Diamond tells us why things like play, sports, music, memorization and reflection are crucial parts of education.

The Body's Grace: Matthew Sanford's Story (October 11, 2007) An unusual take on the mind-body connection with author and yoga teacher Matthew Sanford.

Yoga. Meditation in Action with Seane Corn (September 11, 2008) Seane Corn takes us inside the practicalities and power of yoga.

The "Happiest" Man in the World - Meeting Matthieu Ricard (November 12, 2009) We explore why Buddhist teacher and author Matthieu Ricard been called "the happiest man in the world," and how he understands spirituality as "contemplative science."

The Wisdom of Tenderness (December 20, 2007) Jean Vanier on L'Arche, human touch, and kindness.

Listening Generously: The Medicine of Rachel Naomi Remen (December 27, 2007) Rachel Naomi Remen on listening, healing, and loss helps us live.

The Inner Landscape of Beauty (November 25, 2010) The Irish poet and philosopher John O'Donohue sits down with Krista for a conversation about God and beauty.

Restoring the Senses: Gardening and Orthodox Easter with Vigen Guroian (April 5, 2012) http://being.publicradio.org/programs/2012/restoring-the-senses/ An understanding of Easter from inside the Armenian Orthodox tradition. Vigen Guroian experiences Easter as a call to our senses. He's a theologian who contemplates the grand ideas of incarnation, death, and eternity as they are revealed in life and in his garden.

Laura Kragie, MD: Be the Rainbow • Bridge Heaven and Earth

Opening to Our Lives (January 27, 2011) Jon Kabat-Zinn shares what he has learned about mindfulness as a way of life.

The Power of Eckhart Tolle's Now (August 14, 2008) Eckhart Tolle on spirit and God, pain-bodies, presence, and living with fame.

Science and Hope (May 10, 2007) Quaker George Ellis on ethics and cosmology.

The Science of Trust: Economics and Virtue (July 9, 2009) Pioneering neuroeconomist Paul Zak discusses trust, fair play, empathy, and economics.

The Losses and the Laughter We Grow Into with Kevin Kling (March 15, 2012) Kevin Kling is part funny guy, part poet and playwright, part wise man. Born with a disabled left arm, he lost the use of his right one after a motorcycle accident nearly killed him. He shares his special angle on life's humor and its ruptures — and why we turn loss into story.

OTHER PODCASTS and VIDEOS

Complementary and Alternative Medicine Online Continuing Education Series: http://nccam.nih.gov/training/videolectures/

- Ten Years of Research on Complementary and Alternative Medicine: Promising Ideas from Outside the Mainstream
- Mind-Body Medicine
- Acupuncture: An Evidence-Based Assessment
- Manipulative and Body-Based Therapies: Chiropractic and Spinal Manipulation
- Health and Spirituality
- Neurobiological Correlates of Acupuncture

Herbert Benson: The Relaxation Revolution
http://www.youtube.com/watch?v=cEt9zcsSiK0

Herbert Benson: Steps to Elicit the Relaxation Response

Laura Kragie, MD: Be the Rainbow • Bridge Heaven and Earth

http://www.relaxationresponse.org/steps/

Human Connections Start With A Friendly Touch (Sept 20, 2010)
http://www.npr.org/templates/story/story.php?storyId=128795325

J. Anderson Thomson *Why We Believe in God(s): the Science of Faith*
http://www.youtube.com/watch?v=1iMmvu9eMrg

Is This Your Brain On God? (May19 2009)
http://www.npr.org/templates/story/story.php?storyId=110997741

The Science of the Placebo Effect Luana Colloca MD PhD
http://videocast.nih.gov/launch.asp?16639

RCT and PLACEBO

Daniel E. Moerman, *Physiology and Symbols: The Anthropological Implications of the Placebo Effect* p240: Lola Romanucci-Ross, Daniel E. Moerman (Ed), Laurence R. Tancredi (Ed) **The Anthropology of Medicine: From Culture to Method** 1997 ABC-CLIO, Inc.

Karin Meissner, Niko Kohls and Luana Colloca (Eds.), *Theme issue: Placebo Effects in Medicine: Mechanisms and Clinical Implications* **Phil. Trans. R. Soc. B**. June 27, 2011 366:(1572) 1781-1930

Luana Colloca MD PhD, *The Science of the Placebo Effect*
http://videocast.nih.gov/launch.asp?16639

Andrew Lakoff, *The Right Patients for the Drug: Managing the Placebo Effect in Antidepressant Trials* **BioSocieties** 2007 2:57-71;
doi:10.1017/S174585520700505

60 Minutes, *Treating Depression: Is there a Placebo Effect?* February 19, 2012. A Harvard scientist says the drugs used to treat depression are effective, but for many, it's not the active ingredient that's making people feel better. It's the placebo effect.
http://www.cbsnews.com/video/watch/?id=7399362n&tag=contentBody;
storyMediaBox

Laura Kragie, MD: Be the Rainbow • Bridge Heaven and Earth

Irene Tracey, *Getting the Pain You Expect: Mechanisms of Placebo, Nocebo and Reappraisal Effects in Humans* **Nature Medicine** 2010 Vol 16, Num 11; doi:10.1038/nm.2229 The perception of pain is subject to powerful influences. Understanding how these are mediated at a neuroanatomical and neurobiological level provides us with valuable information that has a direct impact on our ability to harness positive and minimize negative effects therapeutically, as well as optimize clinical trial designs when developing new analgesics. This is particularly relevant for placebo and nocebo effects. New research findings have directly contributed to an increased understanding of how placebo and nocebo effects are produced and what biological and psychological factors influence variances in the magnitude of the effect. The findings have relevance for chronic pain states and other disorders, where abnormal functioning of crucial brain regions might affect analgesic outcome even in the normal therapeutic setting.

Harald O. Stolberg, Geoffrey Norman, Isabelle Trop, *Randomized Controlled Trials* **AJR** 2004; 183:1539-1544. Preceding articles in this series have provided a great deal of information concerning research design and methodology, including research protocols, statistical analyses, and assessment of the clinical importance of radiologic research studies. Many methods of research design have already been presented, including descriptive studies (e.g., case reports, case series, and cross-sectional surveys), and some analytical designs (e.g., cohort and case-control studies). Case-control and cohort studies are also called observational studies, which distinguishes them from interventional (experimental) studies because the decision to seek one treatment or another, or to be exposed to one risk or another, was made by someone other than the experimenter. Consequently, the researcher's role is one of observing the outcome of these exposures. By contrast, in experimental studies, the researcher (experimenter) controls the exposure. The most powerful type of experimental study is the randomized controlled trial. The basic principles of randomized controlled trials will be discussed in this article.

John P. A. Ioannidis, *Why Most Published Research Findings are False* **PLoS Medicine** | www.plosmedicine.org 0696 August 2005 | Volume 2 | Issue 8 | e124 Summary: There is increasing concern that most current published research findings are false. The probability that a research claim is true may depend on study power and bias, the number of other studies on the same question, and, importantly, the ratio of true to no relationships among the relationships probed in each scientific field. In this framework, a research finding is less likely to be true when the studies conducted in a field are smaller; effect sizes are smaller; when there is a greater number and lesser preselection of tested relationships; where there is greater flexibility in designs, definitions, outcomes, and analytical modes; when there is greater financial and other interest and prejudice; and when more teams are involved in a scientific field in chase of statistical significance. Simulations show that for most study designs and settings, it is more likely for a research claim to be false than true. Moreover, for many current scientific fields, claimed research findings may often be simply accurate measures of the prevailing bias. In this essay, I discuss the implications of these problems for the conduct and interpretation of research.

Howard Beckman, Kathryn Markakis, Anthony Suchman, Richard Frankel, *The Doctor-Patient Relationship and Malpractice, Lessons from Plaintiff Depositions* **Arch Intern Med** 1994; 154(12):1365-1370. The decision to litigate was often associated with a perceived lack of caring and/or collaboration in the delivery of health care. The issues identified included perceived unavailability, discounting patient and/or family concerns, poor delivery of information, and lack of understanding the patient and/or family perspective.

CARL GUSTAV JUNG

Carl G. Jung, **The Portable Jung** Joseph Campbell (Ed.), R. F. C. Hull (Trans.) 1976 Penguin. The comprehensive collection of writings by the epoch-shaping Swiss psychoanalyst was edited by Joseph Campbell, himself the most famous of Jung's American followers. It comprises Jung's pioneering studies of the structure of the psyche — including the works that introduced such notions as the collective unconscious, the Shadow, Anima and Animus — as well as inquiries into the psychology of spirituality and creativity, and Jung's influential On Synchronicity, a paper whose implications extend from the I Ching to quantum physics. Campbell's introduction completes this compact volume, placing Jung's astonishingly wide-ranging work within the context of his life and times.

Laura Kragie, MD: Be the Rainbow • Bridge Heaven and Earth

The Power of Myth 1988, an award winning television series featuring Joe Campbell's interviews with Bill Moyers.

Carl G Jung, **The Collected Works** (Bollingen Series XX). (1953-1979) 20 vols. R. F. C. Hull (Trans.). (Ed.) H. Read (Ed.), M. Fordham, G. Adler, Wm. McGuire. Princeton University Press. Jung wrote his essay, *The Transcendent Function* while serving the Swiss military during WWI. Here are some pertinent passages: The process of coming to terms with the unconscious is a true labor, a work that involves both action and suffering. It has been named the "transcendent function" because it represents a function based on real and imaginary, or irrational and rational, data, thus bridging the yawning gulf between conscious and unconscious. It is a natural process, a manifestation of the energy that springs from the tension of opposites, and it consists in a series of fantasy-occurrences that appear spontaneously in dreams and visions. ... When there is full parity of the opposites, attested by the ego's absolute participation in both, this necessarily leads to a suspension of the will, for the will can no longer operate when every motive has an equally strong countermotive. Since life cannot tolerate a standstill, a damming up of vital energy results, and this would lead to an insupportable condition did not the tension of opposites produce a new, uniting function that transcends them. This function arises quite naturally from the regression of libido caused by the blockage. ... The tendencies of the conscious and the unconscious are the two factors that together make up the transcendent function. It is called "transcendent" because it makes the transition from one attitude to another organically possible. Once the unconscious content has been given form and the meaning of the formulation is understood, the question arises as to how the ego will relate to this position, and how the ego and the unconscious are to come to terms. This is the second and more important stage of the procedure, the bringing together of opposites for the production of a third: the transcendent function. At this stage it is no longer the unconscious that takes the lead, but the ego. From the activity of the unconscious there now emerges a new content, constellated by thesis and antithesis in equal measure and standing in a compensatory relation to both. It thus forms the middle ground on which the opposites can be united. If, for instance, we conceive the opposition to be sensuality versus spirituality, then the mediatory content born out of the unconscious provides a welcome means of expression for the spiritual thesis, because of its rich spiritual associations, and also for the sensual antithesis, because of its sensuous imagery. The ego, however, torn between thesis and antithesis, finds in the middle ground its own counterpart, its sole and unique means of expression, and it eagerly seizes on this in order to be delivered from its division. If the mediatory product remains intact, it forms the raw material for a process not of dissolution but of construction, in which thesis and antithesis both play their part. In this way it becomes a new content that governs the whole attitude, putting an end to the division and forcing the energy of the opposites into a common channel. The standstill is overcome and life can flow on with renewed power towards new goals.

WILLIAM JAMES

William James, **The Varieties of Religious Experience** 1902 Modern Library. This book emphasized the validity of subjective, spiritually grounded experiences. Here he criticized "medical materialism that finishes St. Paul by calling his vision on the road to Damascus as a discharging lesion of the occipital cortex" and 'snuffs out St. Theresa as a hysteric." James' response is simple and direct: Believe, if one wishes, by faith — that is, without evidence. James wrote considerably on the concept of pragmatism. According to pragmatism, the truth of an idea can never be proven. James proposed we instead focus on what he called the "cash value," or usefulness, of an idea. James opposed the structuralism focus on introspection and breaking down mental events to the smallest elements. Instead, James focused on the wholeness of an event, taking into the impact of the environment on behavior.

William James, **The Principles of** Psychology 1890 Harvard University Press. The James-Lange theory of emotion proposes that an event triggers a physiological reaction, which we then interpret. According to this theory, emotions are caused by our interpretations of these physiological reactions. Both James and the Danish physiologist Carl Lange independently proposed the theory.

ALBERT EINSTEIN

"The fairest thing we can experience is the mysterious. It is the fundamental emotion which stands at the cradle of true art and true science. He who knows it not and can no longer wonder, no longer feel amazement, is as good as dead, a snuffed-out candle. It was the experience of mystery — even if mixed with fear — that engendered religion. A knowledge of the existence of something we cannot penetrate, of the manifestations of the profoundest reason and the most radiant beauty, which are only accessible to our reason in their most elementary forms — it is this knowledge and this emotion that constitute the truly religious attitude; in this sense, and in this alone, I am a deeply religious man. I cannot conceive of a God who rewards and punishes his creatures, or has a will of the type of which we are conscious in ourselves. An individual who should survive his physical death is also beyond my comprehension, nor do I wish it otherwise; such notions are for the fears or absurd egoism of feeble souls. Enough for me is the mystery of eternity of life, and the inkling of the marvelous structure of reality, together with the single-hearted endeavor to comprehend a portion, be it never so tiny, of the reason that manifests itself in nature." - Albert Einstein

Walter Isaacson, **Einstein: His Life and Universe** 2008 Simon Schuster. "I wanted to capture the imaginative beauty of Einstein's scientific leaps. ... He was actually great in math, because he could visualize equations. He knew they were nature's brushstrokes for painting her wonders. For example, he could look at Maxwell's equations and marvel at what it would be like to ride alongside a light wave, and he could look at Max Planck's equations about radiation and realize that Planck's constant meant that light was a particle as well as a wave." - Walter Isaacson

Krista Tippett, **Einstein's God: Conversations About Science and the Human Spirit** 2010 Penguin. Albert Einstein did not believe in a personal God. And his famous quip that "God does not play dice with the universe" was a statement about quantum physics, not a statement of faith. But he did leave behind a fascinating, largely forgotten legacy of musings and writings — some serious, some whimsical — about the relationship between science and religion and his own inquisitive reverence for the "order deeply hidden behind everything". Einstein's self-described "cosmic religious sense" is intriguingly compatible with twenty-first-century sensibilities. And it is the starting point for Einstein's God. Drawn from American Public Media's extraordinary program *Speaking of Faith*, the conversations in this profoundly illuminating book explore an emerging interface of inquiry — if not answers — between many fields of science, medicine, theology and philosophy. In her interviews with such luminaries as Freeman Dyson, Paul Davies, V. V. Raman, and Mehmet Oz, Krista Tippett draws out the connections between these realms, showing how even those most wedded to hard truths find spiritual enlightenment in the life of experiment and, in turn, raise questions that are richly theologically evocative. Whether she is speaking with celebrated surgeon and author Sherwin Nuland about the biology of the human spirit or questioning Darwin biographer James Moore about his subject's religious beliefs, Tippett offers a rare look at the way our best minds grapple with the questions for which we all seek answers.

COGNITIVE NEUROSCIENCE

Malcolm Gladwell, **Blink: The Power of Thinking Without Thinking** 2005 Little, Brown and Co. In his landmark bestseller **The Tipping Point**, Malcolm Gladwell redefined how we understand the world around us. Now, in **Blink**, he revolutionizes the way we understand the world within. **Blink** is a book about how we think without thinking, about choices that seem to be made in an instant — in the blink of an eye — that actually aren't as simple as they seem. Why are some people brilliant decision makers, while others are consistently inept? Why do some people follow their instincts and win, while others end up stumbling into error? How do our brains really work-in the office, in the classroom, in the kitchen, and in the bedroom? And why are the best decisions often those that are impossible to explain to others? In Blink we meet the psychologist who has learned to predict whether a marriage will last, based on a few minutes of observing a couple; the tennis coach who knows when a player will double-fault before the racket even makes contact with the ball; the antiquities experts who recognize a fake at a glance. Here, too, are great failures of "blink": the election of Warren Harding; "New Coke"; and the shooting of Amadou Diallo by police. Blink reveals that great decision makers aren't those who process the most information or spend the most time deliberating, but those who have perfected the art of "thin-slicing"—filtering the very few factors that matter from an overwhelming number of variables.

V. S. Ramachandran, Sandra Blakeslee, Oliver Sacks (Fwd), **Phantoms in the Brain: Probing the Mysteries of the Human Mind** 1998 Harper. Neuroscientist Ramachandran is internationally renowned for uncovering answers to the deep and quirky questions of human nature that few scientists have dared to address. His bold insights about the brain are matched only by the stunning simplicity of his experiments — using such low-tech tools as cotton swabs, glasses of water and dime-store mirrors. In **Phantoms in the Brain**, he recounts how his work with patients who have bizarre neurological disorders has shed new light on the deep architecture of the brain, and what these findings tell us about who we are, how we construct our body image, why we laugh or become depressed, why we may believe in God, how we make decisions, deceive ourselves and dream, perhaps even why we're so clever at philosophy, music and art. Some of his most notable cases: A woman paralyzed on the left side of her body who believes she is lifting a tray of drinks with both hands offers a unique opportunity to test Freud's theory of denial. A man who insists he is talking with God challenges us to ask: Could we be "wired" for religious experience? A woman who hallucinates cartoon characters illustrates how, in a sense, we are all hallucinating, all the time. Dr. Ramachandran's inspired medical detective work pushes the boundaries of medicine's last great frontier — the human mind — yielding new and provocative insights into the "big questions" about consciousness and the self. See also: http://ajp.psychiatryonline.org/article.aspx?Volume=157&page=841&journalID=13

Christof Koch, **The Quest for Consciousness: A Neurobiological Approach** 2004 Roberts and Co. In this book Caltech neuroscientist Christof Koch explores the biological basis of consciousness. He outlines a framework that he and Francis Crick have constructed to come to grips with the ancient mind-body problem. At the heart of their framework is a sustained, empirical approach to discovering and characterizing the neuronal correlates of consciousness—the NCC — the subtle, flickering patterns of brain activity that underlie each and every conscious experience.

Antonio R. Damasio, **Descartes' Error: Emotion, Reason, and the Human Brain** 1994 Penguin. In this wondrously lucid and engaging book, renowned neurologist Antonio Damasio demonstrates what many of us have long suspected: emotions are not a luxury, they are essential to rational thinking. Descartes' Error takes the reader on an enthralling journey of scientific discovery, starting with the case of Phineas Gage — a construction foreman who in 1848 survived a freak accident in which a 3 1/2 foot iron rod passed through his head — and continuing on to Damasio's experiences with modern-day neurological patients affected by brain damage. Far from interfering with rationality, his research shows us, the absence of emotion and feeling can break down rationality and make wise decision making almost impossible.

David Eagleman, **Incognito: The Secret Lives of the Brain** 2011 Pantheon. If the conscious mind — the part you consider you — is just the tip of the iceberg in the brain, what is all the rest doing? Neuroscientist Eagleman plumbs the depths of the subconscious brain to illuminate surprising questions: Why can your foot jump halfway to the brake pedal before you become consciously aware of danger ahead? Why do strippers make more money at certain times of month, even while no one is consciously aware of their fertility level? Is there a true Mel Gibson? What do Odysseus and the subprime mortgage meltdown have in common? How is your brain like a conflicted democracy engaged in civil war? Why are people whose name begins with J more likely to marry other people whose name begins with J? Why is it so difficult to keep a secret? Why did Supreme Court Justice William Douglas deny that he was paralyzed? The subsurface exploration includes waystops in brain damage, drugs, infidelity, synesthesia, criminal law, the future of artificial intelligence, and visual illusions — all highlighting how our perception of the world is a hidden and awe-inspiring construction of the brain.

Jonah Lehrer, **How We Decide** 2009 Houghton Mifflin Harcourt. Since Plato, philosophers have described the decision-making process as either rational or emotional: we carefully deliberate or we "blink" and go with our gut. But as scientists break open the mind's black box with the latest tools of neuroscience, they're discovering that this is not how the mind works. Our best decisions are a finely tuned blend of both feeling and reason — and the precise mix depends on the situation. When buying a house, for example, it's best to let our unconscious mull over the many variables. But when we're picking a stock, intuition often leads us astray. The trick is to determine when to lean on which part of the brain, and to do this, we need to think harder (and smarter) about how we think. Jonah Lehrer arms us with the tools we need, drawing on cutting-edge research by Daniel Kahneman, Colin Camerer, and others, as well as the real-world experiences of a wide range of "deciders" — from airplane pilots and hedge fund investors to serial killers and poker players. Lehrer shows how people are taking advantage of the new science to make better television shows, win more football games, and improve military intelligence. His goal is to answer two questions that are of interest to just about anyone, from CEOs to firefighters: How does the human mind make decisions? And how can we make those decisions better?

Jonah Lehrer, **Imagine: How Creativity Works** 2012 Houghton Mifflin Harcourt. Did you know that the most creative companies have centralized bathrooms? That brainstorming meetings are a terrible idea? That the color blue can help you double your creative output? From the New York Times best-selling author of **How We Decide** comes a sparkling and revelatory look at the new science of creativity. Shattering the myth of muses, higher powers, even creative "types," Jonah Lehrer demonstrates that creativity is not a single gift possessed by the lucky few. It's a variety of distinct thought processes that we can all learn to use more effectively. Lehrer reveals the importance of embracing the rut, thinking like a child, daydreaming productively, and adopting an outsider's perspective (travel helps). He unveils the optimal mix of old and new partners in any creative collaboration, and explains why criticism is essential to the process. Then he zooms out to show how we can make our neighborhoods more vibrant, our companies more productive, and our schools more effective. You'll learn about Bob Dylan's writing habits and the drug addictions of poets. You'll meet a Manhattan bartender who thinks like a chemist, and an autistic surfer who invented an entirely new surfing move. You'll see why Elizabethan England experienced a creative explosion, and how Pixar's office space is designed to spark the next big leap in animation. Collapsing the layers separating the neuron from the finished symphony, Imagine reveals the deep inventiveness of the human mind, and its essential role in our increasingly complex world.

David Linden, **The Compass of Pleasure: How Our Brains Make Fatty Foods, Orgasm, Exercise, Marijuana, Generosity, Vodka, Learning, and Gambling Feel So Good** 2011 Viking. In his book, neurobiologist David Linden explicates the workings of these [brain] regions, known collectively as the reward system, elegantly drawing on sources ranging from personal experience to studies of brain activity to experiments with molecules and genes. Linden builds a powerful case that every kind of substance, activity or stimulus that motivates human choice does so because it acts on this particular network, whose neurons use the chemical dopamine to communicate with one another. - The **New York Times** *Book Review*

Daniel Kahneman, **Thinking, Fast and Slow** 2011 Macmillan. Daniel Kahneman, recipient of the Nobel Prize in Economic Sciences for his seminal work in psychology that challenged the rational model of judgment and decision making, is one of our most important thinkers. His ideas have had a profound and widely regarded impact on many fields — including economics, medicine, and politics—but until now, he has never brought together his many years of research and thinking in one book. In the highly anticipated book, Kahneman takes us on a groundbreaking tour of the mind and explains the two systems that drive the way we think. System 1 is fast, intuitive, and emotional; System 2 is slower, more deliberative, and more logical. Kahneman exposes the extraordinary capabilities — and also the faults and biases — of fast thinking, and reveals the pervasive influence of intuitive impressions on our thoughts and behavior. The impact of loss aversion and overconfidence on corporate strategies, the difficulties of predicting what will make us happy in the future, the challenges of properly framing risks at work and at home, the profound effect of cognitive biases on everything from playing the stock market to planning the next vacation — each of these can be understood only by knowing how the two systems work together to shape our judgments and decisions. Engaging the reader in a lively conversation about how we think, Kahneman reveals where we can and cannot trust our intuitions and how we can tap into the benefits of slow thinking. He offers practical and enlightening insights into how choices are made in both our business and our personal lives — and how we can use different techniques to guard against the mental glitches that often get us into trouble. **Thinking, Fast and Slow** will transform the way you think about thinking. As the psychologist Daniel Gilbert has observed, disbelieving is hard work.

Joshua Foer, **Moonwalking with Einstein: The Art and Science of Remembering Everything** 2011 Penguin. Foer found a vital truth we too often forget: in every way that matters, we are the sum of our memories. This book draws on cutting-edge research, a surprising cultural history of memory, and venerable tricks of the mentalist's trade to transform our understanding of human remembering. Immersing himself obsessively in a quirky subculture of competitive memorizers, Foer learns to apply techniques that call on imagination as much as determination-showing that memorization can be anything but rote. From the PAO system, which converts numbers into lurid images, to the memory palace, in which memories are stored in the rooms of imaginary structures, Foer's experience shows that the World Memory Championships are less a test of memory than of perseverance and creativity. "The 'art' is in creating imagery in your mind that is so unusual, so colorful, so unlike anything you've ever seen before that it's unlikely to be forgotten. That's why mnemonists like to say that their skills are as much about creativity as memory … The OK Plateau is that place we all get to where we just stop getting better at something. Take typing, for example. You might type and type and type all day long, but once you reach a certain level, you just never get appreciably faster at it. That's because it's become automatic. You've moved it to the back of your mind's filing cabinet. If you want to become a faster typer, it's possible, of course. But you've got to bring the task back under your conscious control." - Joshua Foer

Michael Shermer, **The Believing Brain: From Ghosts and Gods to Politics and Conspiracies — How We Construct Beliefs and Reinforce Them as Truths** 2011 Times Books. Lucidly describes why and how we are hard wired to 'want to believe'. Simply put, beliefs come first and explanations for beliefs follow. The brain, Shermer argues, is a belief engine. From sensory data flowing in through the senses, the brain naturally begins to look for and find patterns, and then infuses those patterns with meaning. Our brains connect the dots of our world into meaningful patterns that explain why things happen, and these patterns become beliefs. Once beliefs are formed the brain begins to look for and find confirmatory evidence in support of those beliefs, which accelerates the process of reinforcing them, and round and round the process goes in a positive-feedback loop of belief confirmation. Shermer outlines the numerous cognitive tools our brains engage to reinforce our beliefs as truths.

Laura Kragie, MD: Be the Rainbow • Bridge Heaven and Earth

David Brooks, **Social Animal: The Hidden Sources of Love, Character, and Achievement** 2011 Random House. With the intellectual curiosity and emotional wisdom that make his columns among the most read in the nation, Brooks turns to the building blocks of human flourishing in a multilayered, profoundly illuminating work grounded in everyday life. This is the story of how success happens. It is told through the lives of one composite American couple, Harold and Erica — how they grow, push forward, are pulled back, fail, and succeed. Distilling a vast array of information into these two vividly realized characters, Brooks illustrates a fundamental new understanding of human nature. A scientific revolution has occurred — we have learned more about the human brain in the last thirty years than we had in the previous three thousand. The unconscious mind, it turns out, is most of the mind — not a dark, vestigial place but a creative and enchanted one, where most of the brain's work gets done. This is the realm of emotions, intuitions, biases, longings, genetic predispositions, personality traits, and social norms: the realm where character is formed and where our most important life decisions are made. The natural habitat of **The Social Animal**. Drawing on a wealth of current research from numerous disciplines, Brooks takes Harold and Erica from infancy to school; from the "odyssey years" that have come to define young adulthood to the high walls of poverty; from the nature of attachment, love, and commitment, to the nature of effective leadership. He reveals the deeply social aspect of our very minds and exposes the bias in modern culture that overemphasizes rationalism, individualism, and IQ. Along the way, he demolishes conventional definitions of success while looking toward a culture based on trust and humility. **The Social Animal** is a moving and nuanced intellectual adventure, a story of achievement and a defense of progress. Impossible to put down, it is an essential book for our time, one that will have broad social impact and will change the way we see ourselves and the world.

Nicholas Christakis, James Fowler, **Connected: The Surprising Power of Our Social Networks and How They Shape Our Lives** 2009 Little, Brown and Co. Harvard professor and health care policy specialist Christakis became interested in social connectivity when observing that the mortality rate of spouses spike after a partner passes away. Christakis sought out a collaboration with Fowler, a health systems and political scientist, and together they compare topology (the hows of a given structure) across different social networks to better explain how participation and positioning enhances the effectiveness of an individual, and why the "whole" of a network is "greater than the sum of its parts." Five basic rules describe the relationship between individuals and their networks — including mutual adaptation, the influence of friends and friends' friends, the network's "life of its own"— but the results do more than promote the good of the group: they also spread contagions; create "epidemics" of obesity, smoking and substance abuse; disseminate fads and markets; alter voting patterns; and more. A thorough but popular take on a complex phenomenon, this volume offers an entertaining guide to the mechanics and importance of human networking.

Vanderbilt University (2011, July 19). *Memories may skew visual perception*. ScienceDaily. http://www.sciencedaily.com/releases/2011/07/110720091542.htm "There are numerous instances where we engage in visually guided activities, such as driving, while rehashing visual events in our mind's eye. Common sense tells us that this mental replay is harmless in that it does not interfere with our ability to register and react to objects within our visual field," Kang and his co-authors wrote. "Evidently, however, that is not always true when the contents of our working memories overlap with the contents of our perceptual world." "We find that observers misperceive the actual direction of motion of a single motion stimulus if, while viewing that stimulus, they are holding a different motion direction in visual working memory. Holding the memory of a visual event in our mind for a short period of time can 'contaminate' visual perception during the time that we're remembering," Randolph Blake, study co-author and Centennial Professor of Psychology, said. "Our study represents the first conclusive evidence for such contamination, and the results strongly suggest that remembering and perceiving engage at least some of the same brain areas."

It happens with numbers too:

Association for Psychological Science (2011, July 20). *Time and numbers mix together in the brain*. ScienceDaily. http://www.sciencedaily.com-/releases/2011/07/110719171549.htm People associate small numbers with short time intervals and large numbers with longer intervals. The influence of the digit is so automatic and so immediate," Wu says. "The results suggest that the brain somehow processes time and the size of numbers together — possibly even with the same neurons. So, maybe instead of having different parts of the brain devoted to different kinds of measurement, there's some part of the brain that is generally responsible for thinking about magnitude. It shows that it's not like, mentally, we have a clock and it is immune to all the other information," Wu says. Instead, your concept of time is responding to other things going on in the brain. In this case, it's numbers, but it might also be influenced by emotion. For example, we all know that time passes more slowly in a boring meeting than when you're chatting with a friend; maybe this is related to the ways that timekeeping links to other functions in the brain.

MUSIC THERAPY

Oliver Sacks, **Musicophilia: Tales of Music and the Brain** 2007 Knopf. Music can move us to the heights or depths of emotion. It can persuade us to buy something, or remind us of our first date. It can lift us out of depression when nothing else can. It can get us dancing to its beat. But the power of music goes much, much further. Indeed, music occupies more areas of our brain than language does — humans are a musical species. Oliver Sacks's compassionate, compelling tales of people struggling to adapt to different neurological conditions have fundamentally changed the way we think of our own brains, and of the human experience. In **Musicophilia** he examines the powers of music through the individual experiences of patients, musicians, and everyday people — from a man who is struck by lightning and suddenly inspired to become a pianist at the age of forty-two, to an entire group of children with Williams syndrome, who are hypermusical from birth; from people with "amusia," to whom a symphony sounds like the clattering of pots and pans, to a man whose memory spans only seven seconds — for everything but music. Our exquisite sensitivity to music can sometimes go wrong: Sacks explores how catchy tunes can subject us to hours of mental replay, and how a surprising number of people acquire nonstop musical hallucinations that assault them night and day. Yet far more frequently, music goes right: Sacks describes how music can animate people with Parkinson's disease who cannot otherwise move, give words to stroke patients who cannot otherwise speak, and calm and organize people whose memories are ravaged by Alzheimer's or amnesia. Music is irresistible, haunting, and unforgettable, and in

Laura Kragie, MD: Be the Rainbow • Bridge Heaven and Earth

Musicophilia, Oliver Sacks tells us why.

NPR Science Friday with Ira Flatow (December 15 2011) *Music Therapy Singing for Pain*
http://www.sciencefriday.com/program/archives/201112161 Treating Stress, Speech Disorders With Music: More and more hospitals and clinics now offer music therapy as a supplementary treatment for everything from anxiety to Alzheimer's, but its efficacy varies for different conditions. Neurologist Oliver Sacks and several music therapists discuss the science and practice of music therapy.

Mary Ishimoto Morris, *Therapeutic Music Aims to Ease the Pain for the Seriously Ill* (December 23, 2008) http://www.washingtonpost.com/wp-dyn/content/article/2008/12/19/AR2008121903041.html?hpid=sec-health

Daniel Levitin, **The World in Six Songs How the Musical Brain Created Human Nature** 2009 Penguin. The author of **This Is Your Brain on Music** tunes us in to six evolutionary musical forms that brought about the evolution of human culture. An unprecedented blend of science and art, Daniel Levitin's debut, **This Is Your Brain on Music**, delighted readers with an exuberant guide to the neural impulses behind those songs that make our heart swell. Now he showcases his daring theory of "six songs," illuminating how the brain evolved to play and listen to music in six fundamental forms — for knowledge, friendship, religion, joy, comfort, and love. Preserving the emotional history of our lives and of our species, from its very beginning music was also allied to dance, as the structure of the brain confirms; developing this neurological observation, Levitin shows how music and dance enabled the social bonding and friendship necessary for human culture and society to evolve. Blending cutting-edge scientific findings with his own sometimes hilarious experiences as a musician and music-industry professional, Levitin's sweeping study also incorporates wisdom gleaned from interviews with icons ranging from Sting and Paul Simon to Joni Mitchell, and David Byrne, along with classical musicians and conductors, historians, anthropologists, and evolutionary biologists. The result is a brilliant revelation of the prehistoric yet elegant systems at play when we sing and dance at a wedding or cheer at a concert — or tune out quietly with an iPod.

Laura Kragie, MD: Be the Rainbow • Bridge Heaven and Earth

Michaeleen Doucleff, *Anatomy of a Tear-Jerker: Why does Adele's 'Someone Like You' make everyone cry? Science has found the formula.* February 11, 2012 WSJ.com http://online.wsj.com/article/SB10001424052970203646004577213010291701378.html An appoggiatura is a type of ornamental note that clashes with the melody just enough to create a dissonant sound. "This generates tension in the listener," said Martin Guhn, a psychologist who co-wrote a 2007 study on the subject. "When the notes return to the anticipated melody, the tension resolves, and it feels good." Chills often descend on listeners at these moments of resolution.

On the Media: *How Music Conveys Emotion* (February 17, 2012) http://www.onthemedia.org/2012/feb/17/how-music-conveys-emotion/ Adele won best pop solo performance Grammy for her song Someone Like You. To learn how music conveys emotion, we talked to McGill professor Dan Levitin about what makes music, and in particular Adele's *Someone Like You*, so emotionally powerful.

Soundcheck® *The Healing Power of Music* http://www.wnyc.org/shows/soundcheck/2009/aug/24/the-healing-power-of-music/ A group of wounded veterans are playing death metal and composing rap lyrics as part of their rehabilitation at Walter Reed Army Medical Center. Eclectic composer Arthur Bloom joins us to tell us the story of a program called MusiCorps. And we ask neuroscientist, cognitive psychologist, and former record producer Daniel Levitin about the role of music in physical and psychological healing.

RELAXATION RESPONSE

Herbert Benson, William Proctor, **Relaxation Revolution** 2010 Simon and Shuster. When Dr. Herbert Benson introduced this simple, effective, mind/body approach to relieve stress in **The Relaxation Response** twenty-five years ago, the book became an instant national bestseller. Since that time, millions of people have learned the secret of the relaxation response — without high-priced lectures, drugs, or prescription medicine. The tremendous success of this approach has turned **The Relaxation Response** into the classic reference recommended by most health care professionals and authorities to treat the harmful effects of stress. This revitalizing, therapeutic approach, discovered by Dr. Benson and his colleagues, is now routinely recommended to treat patients suffering from heart conditions, high blood pressure, chronic pain, insomnia, and many other physical ailments. Requiring only minutes to learn, and just ten to twenty minutes of practice twice a day, the Relaxation Response has proven to be one of the most effective ways to relieve the tensions of modern-day living for a richer, healthier, more productive life. Recent scientific breakthroughs demonstrating that mind body strategies can actually "switch off" or "switch on" gene activity associated with health and disease have triggered a mind body revolution in the medical world. In the 1970s, Dr. Herbert Benson of Harvard Medical School ushered in a new era of understanding in the field of mind body medicine. Coining the term "relaxation response," Dr. Benson identified the body's physiologic reaction that is the exact opposite of the stress (fight-or-flight) response. In the four decades since that initial discovery, Benson and his colleagues have established effective therapy to counteract the harmful effects of stress. They have explored how the relaxation response, the power of expectation and belief, and other mind body phenomena can produce healing in your own body. **Relaxation Revolution** details Dr. Benson's recent work with colleagues in the field of genetics, which links mind body treatments to the healing of a steadily expanding number of medical conditions. Mind and body have become part of a scientific and medical whole; together they represent a complete approach to healing and maximal well-being. In clear, straightforward language, Benson and Proctor cite the experiences of real people to show how mind body techniques have the potential not only to enhance healing but also to reduce health costs to individuals and to society as a whole. See also:

Herbert Benson: The Relaxation Revolution
http://www.youtube.com/watch?v=cEt9zcsSiK0

Herbert Benson: Steps to Elicit the Relaxation Response
http://www.relaxationresponse.org/steps/

James Nestor, **Get High Now** 2009 Chronicle Books. This book is an illustrated, mind-blowing magic carpet ride of more than 175 ways to alter human perception and consciousness — without drugs or alcohol. Based on science — not subjective New Age hearsay — **Get High Now** explores the worlds of neurology, biology, and physiology through meditations, illusions, common herbs, audio and visual stimulations, and some bizarre anthropological discoveries. Each entry describes in colorful detail how these highs affect our minds and bodies, as well as step-by-step directions for how to do them. Highs include: Breathing Meditations (Indian yogis have been going out-of-body with breath work for millennia); Audio Entrainment (Audio loops discovered in 1839 trick the hemispheres in your brain to hallucinate a three-dimensional tone between your eyes); Cheese (A 2007 British study showed 67 percent of people who ate one ounce of certain cheeses before bed reported wild, fantastical, and sometimes life-changing lucid dreams); Insects (Brazilian bamboo moth larva is a powerful narcotic and multiple bee stings lead to intense hallucinations); Self-Hypnotism (Einstein and Thomas Edison used hypnagogia to think-up their most famous inventions. It's as easy as holding up your arm); Kitchen Herbs (Norse Vikings went berserk off rosemary; dill soothes the mind; eating basil relieves headaches); Animals (Tribes in Sudan hunt the giraffe and drink its liver to induce spiritual visions; the blood of schizophrenics contain the same psychotropic chemical found in hallucinogenic toads and in some Russian reindeer urine ... and so damn many more.)

Julie Rovner, *Pet Therapy: How Animals And Humans Heal Each Other* http://www.npr.org/blogs/health/2012/03/05/146583986/pet-therapy-how-animals-and-humans-heal-each-other Those of us who own pets know they make us happy. But a growing body of scientific research is showing that our pets can also make us healthy, or healthier. That helps explain the increasing use of animals — dogs and cats mostly, but also birds, fish and even horses — in settings ranging from hospitals and nursing homes to schools, jails and mental institutions.

EMBODIMENT

Mark Johnson, **The Body In The Mind: The Bodily Basis Of Meaning, Imagination, and Reason** 1987 University of Chicago Press. Explores the ways that meaning, understanding, and rationality arise from and are conditioned by the patterns of our bodily experience. In emphasizing the role of the body, Mark Johnson offers a corrective to dominant theories of meaning in Western philosophy, which have maintained a strictly abstract, propositional account of meaning detached from persons or experience. Expanding on his work with George Lakoff in the pathbreaking book

Laura Kragie, MD: Be the Rainbow • Bridge Heaven and Earth

Metaphors We Live By Johnson presents here an extended philosophical account, exposing the inadequacies of the objectivist philosophical tradition in its rigid separation of mind from body, cognition from emotion, and reason from imagination. He develops a constructive theory of the ways in which imagination links cognitive and bodily structures.

Mark Johnson, **The Meaning of the Body: Aesthetics of Human Understanding** 2007 University of Chicago. Mark Johnson continues his pioneering work on the exciting connections between cognitive science, language, and meaning first begun in the classic **Metaphors We Live By**. Johnson uses recent research into infant psychology to show how the body generates meaning even before self-consciousness has fully developed. From there he turns to cognitive neuroscience to further explore the bodily origins of meaning, thought, and language and examines the many dimensions of meaning — including images, qualities, emotions, and metaphors — that are all rooted in the body's physical encounters with the world. Drawing on the psychology of art and pragmatist philosophy, Johnson argues that all of these aspects of meaning-making are fundamentally aesthetic. He concludes that the arts are the culmination of human attempts to find meaning and that studying the aesthetic dimensions of our experience is crucial to unlocking meaning's bodily sources. Throughout, Johnson puts forth a bold new conception of the mind rooted in the understanding that philosophy will matter to nonphilosophers only if it is built on a visceral connection to the world.

Simon Lacey, Randall Stilla, K. Sathian, *Metaphorically Feeling: Comprehending Textural Metaphors Activates Somatosensory Cortex Brain and Language*, 2012; DOI: 10.1016/j.bandl.2011.12.016 Linguists and psychologists have debated how much the parts of the brain that mediate direct sensory experience are involved in understanding metaphors. George Lakoff and Mark Johnson, in their landmark work **Metaphors We Live By**, pointed out that our daily language is full of metaphors, some of which are so familiar (like "rough day") that they may not seem especially novel or striking. They argued that metaphor comprehension is grounded in our sensory and motor experiences. New brain imaging research reveals that a region of the brain important for sensing texture through touch, the parietal operculum, is also activated when someone listens to a sentence with a textural metaphor. The same region is not activated when a similar sentence expressing the meaning of the metaphor is heard. We see that metaphors are engaging the areas of the cerebral cortex involved in sensory responses even though the metaphors are quite familiar," says senior author Krish Sathian, MD, PhD. "This result illustrates how we draw upon sensory experiences to achieve understanding of metaphorical language." Visual cortical regions were not activated by textural metaphors, which fits with other evidence for the primacy of touch in texture perception," says Simon Lacey, PhD. The researchers did not find metaphor-specific differences in cortical regions well known to be involved in generating and processing language, such as Broca's or Wernicke's areas. The brain is conducting an internal simulation as a way to understand the metaphor, and that's why the regions associated with touch get involved. This demonstrates how complex processes involving symbols, such as appreciating a painting or understanding a metaphor, do not depend just on evolutionarily new parts of the brain, but also on adaptations of older parts of the brain."

University of Groningen, *If You Don't Show Your Disgust, Your Emotions May Stay Negative.* ScienceDaily (2009, March 18) http://www.sciencedaily.com/releases/2009/03/090312093916.htm Suppression of your disgust, in particular, has negative consequences, even in people who are not aware that they are no longer capable of expressing it 'because their facial muscles have been paralysed by a botox treatment, for example'. People who are able and do express their disgust, feel this emotion more intensely for a short period and then think a lot about related subjects. 'However', says Grob, 'when they find themselves in a new situation, the feeling has completely disappeared. This means that they are no longer bothered by it'. Subjects who were asked to suppress their disgust when shown images of, for example, a dirty toilet or a film depicting an amputation, were able to do so. 'But the emotion then found its way into the open through other channels', says Grob. 'At the cognitive level, they began to think about disgusting things much more often and also felt much more negatively about other issues. People who view the world with negative eyes experience more negative emotions. 'If they also suppress these emotions, they will soon enter a negative spiral. This is something to take into account in a society where more and more people allow their facial muscles to be paralysed by botox treatments for the sake of beauty. This negative spiral is evident with both conscious and unconscious suppression.'

Laura Kragie, MD: Be the Rainbow • Bridge Heaven and Earth

Ivan Norscia, Elisabetta Palagi, *Yawn Contagion and Empathy in Homo sapiens.* PLoS ONE, 2011; 6 (12): e28472 DOI: 10.1371/journal.pone.0028472 Everybody knows that yawning is contagious. When a person yawns, other people can respond by yawning. What wasn't known is that "yawn transmission" is more frequent, and faster, between people sharing an empathic bond: close friends, kin, and mates. The study carried out by Ivan Norscia and Elisabetta Palagi provides the first behavioural evidence that yawn infectiveness can be a form of emotional contagion. "What appears to be most important in affecting contagion is the relationship quality that links the yawner to the 'yawnee'. It is, in fact, more likely that a person "yawn back" if the first yawner is a loved one. A yawn can be a sign of empathy.

Randy Dotinga, HealthDay 06/23/10 June 2010 **Emotion** For Botox users concerned that the muscle-paralyzing injections will rob their face of its ability to show emotion, a new study suggests that people injected with the toxin might end up with less strong emotion to display in the first place. Researchers at Barnard College found that facial expressions appear to play a role in how your emotions develop, not just in how you display them for others to see. The study suggests that facial expressions themselves may influence emotional experiences through a kind of feedback loop. In short, Botox — a toxin that weakens or paralyzes muscles — not only changes one's appearance, but also appears to deaden real emotions. "In a bigger picture sense, the work fits with common beliefs, such as 'fake it till you make it,'" study co-author Joshua Davis said. "With the advent of Botox, it is now possible to work with people who have a temporary, reversible paralysis in muscles that are involved in facial expressions. The muscle paralysis allows us to isolate the effects of facial expression and the subsequent sensory feedback to the brain that would follow from other factors, such as intentions relating to one's expressions, and motor commands to make an expression." Davis explained that "with Botox, a person can respond otherwise normally to an emotional event, e.g., a sad movie scene, but will have less movement in the facial muscles that have been injected, and therefore less feedback to the brain about such facial expressivity. It thus allows for a test of whether facial expressions and the sensory feedback from them to the brain can influence our emotions."

Wolfgang Tschacher, Steven Greenwood, Volker Kirchberg, Stéphanie

Laura Kragie, MD: Be the Rainbow • Bridge Heaven and Earth

Wintzerith, Karen van den Berg, Martin Tröndle, *Physiological Correlates of Aesthetic Perception of Artworks in a Museum.* **Psychology of Aesthetics, Creativity, and the Arts** Jul 18, 2011, doi: 10.1037/a0023845 Abstract: Arts experts are commonly skeptical of applying scientific methods to aesthetic experiencing, which remains a field of study predominantly for the humanities. Laboratory research has, however, indicated that artworks may elicit emotional and physiological responses. Yet, this line of aesthetics research has previously suffered from insufficient external validity. We, therefore, conducted a study in which aesthetic perception was monitored in a fine art museum, unrestricting to the viewers' freedom of aesthetic choice. Visitors were invited to wear electronic gloves through which their locomotion, heart rate and skin conductance were continuously recorded. Emotional and aesthetic responses to selected works of an exhibition were assessed using a customized questionnaire. In a sample of 373 adult participants, we found that physiological responses during perception of an artwork were significantly related to aesthetic-emotional experiencing. The dimensions "Aesthetic Quality," "Surprise / Humor," "Dominance," and "Curatorial Quality" were associated with cardiac measures (heart rate variability, heart rate level) and skin conductance variability. This is the first evidence that aesthetics can be statistically grounded in viewers' physiology in an ecologically valid environment — the art gallery — enhancing our understanding of the effects of artworks and their curatorial staging. The conclusion: an aesthetic appreciation of artwork creates a physical as well as an emotional reaction.

Paul Eckman, **Emotions Revealed: Recognizing Faces and Feelings to Improve Communication and Emotional Life** 2nd Ed 2007 Holt Paperbacks. Renowned psychologist Paul Ekman explains the roots of our emotions — anger, fear, disgust, sadness, and happiness — and shows how they cascade across our faces, providing clear signals to those who can identify the clues. As featured in Malcolm Gladwell's bestseller **Blink**, Ekman's Facial Action Coding System offers intense training in recognizing feelings in spouses, children, colleagues, even strangers on the street. In **Emotions Revealed**, Ekman distills decades of research into a practical, mind-opening, and life-changing guide to reading the emotions of those around us. He answers such questions as: How does our body signal to others whether we are slightly sad or anguished, peeved or enraged? Can we learn to distinguish between a polite smile and the genuine thing? Can we ever truly control our emotions? Packed with unique exercises and photographs, and a new chapter on emotions and lying that encompasses security and terrorism as well as gut decisions, **Emotions Revealed** is an indispensable resource for navigating our emotional world.

John Cloud, *Beyond Drugs; Touch and Pain* **TIME** Mar. 11, 2011 http://www.time.com/time/specials/packages/article/0,28804,2053382_2 055269_2055260-2,00.htm Touching your hand reduces pain from burn. Simple touch can minimize complex central pain. They used a method called the thermal-grill illusion to prove their point. The thermal-grill illusion was a quirky choice because it is best known as a 19th century carnival act. Subjects are asked to touch a very warm object — say, a heated but not scorching grill — and then, right afterward, a cool or room-temperature grill. Quite reliably, the participants' brains fool them into believing the second object is excruciatingly hot, even though nothing has happened to their flesh. Today we know that burning sensation as central pain. The Current Biology team replicated the illusion in a lab experiment using water. Study participants immersed their index and ring fingers in 109°F (39°C) water and their middle fingers in 57°F (14°C) water. As in the original illusion, their middle fingers felt significantly hotter than they really were. The scientists then had participants repeat the experiment with their right fingers only. Immediately after, the subjects used the same three fingers on their left hand to touch the wet fingers on the right hand. This mere touch caused a 64% reduction in self-reported pain scores on a scale of 1 to 100.

William J. Broad, **The Science of Yoga: The Risks and Rewards** 2012 Simon & Schuster. In this remarkable book about yoga, William Broad, a lifelong practitioner, shows us that uncommon states are integral to a hidden world of risk and reward that lies beneath clouds of myth, superstition, and hype. Five years in the making, **The Science of Yoga** draws on more than a century of painstaking research to present the first impartial evaluation of a practice thousands of years old. It celebrates what's real and shows what's illusory, describes what's uplifting and beneficial and what's flaky and dangerous — and why. Broad illuminates how yoga can lift moods and inspire creativity. He exposes moves that can cripple and kill. As science often does, this groundbreaking book also reveals mysteries. It presents a fascinating body of evidence that raises questions about whether humans have latent capabilities for entering states of suspended animation and unremitting sexual bliss. The **Science of Yoga** takes us on a riveting tour of unknown yoga that goes from old archives in Calcutta to the world capitals of medical research, from storied ashrams to spotless laboratories, from sweaty yoga studios with master teachers to the cozy offices of yoga healers. Broad unveils a burgeoning global industry that attracts not only curious scientists but true believers and charismatic hustlers. In the end, he shatters myths, lays out unexpected benefits, and offers a compelling vision of how the ancient practice can be improved.

Eileen Rivers, *A Breath of Hope: Walter Reed Tries Yoga to Counter PTSD* Washington Post Tuesday, May 6, 2008; Page HE01. Describes the success of a program to introduce meditation and yoga practices to incoming wounded soldiers trying to recover from Post Traumatic Stress Disorder.

L.A. Rhodes, C.A. McPhillips-Tangum, C. Markham, R. Klenk, 1999 *The Power of the Visible: the Meaning of Diagnostic Tests in Chronic Back Pain* **Social Science and Medicine** 48: (9) 1189–203. This article explores the meaning of diagnostic tests for people with chronic back pain. Lower back pain is one of the most common health problems in the US. Five to ten percent of the patients who visit a primary care provider for back pain ultimately develop a chronic condition. We draw on interviews with chronic back pain patients in Atlanta, Dallas and Seattle to argue that testing constitutes an important element in the legitimation of pain for these patients. We discuss three aspects that make testing an area of concern for patients: a strong historical connection between visual images and the medicalization of the interior of the body, a set of cultural assumptions that make seeing into the body central to confirming and normalizing patients' symptoms, and the concreteness of diagnostic images themselves. Our interviews show that when physicians cannot locate the problem or express doubt about the possibility of a solution, patients feel that their pain is disconfirmed. Faced with the disjunction between the cultural model of the visible body and the private experience of pain, patients are alienated not only from individual physicians but from an important aspect of the symbolic world of medicine. This paper concludes by suggesting that a fluid, less localized understanding of pain could provide a greater sense of legitimacy for back pain patients.

Laura Kragie, MD: Be the Rainbow • Bridge Heaven and Earth

Jennifer Tarr, *Educating with the Hands: Working on the Body / Self in Alexander Technique* **Sociology of Health & Illness** 2011 ISSN 0141–9889, pp. 1–14 doi: 10.1111/j.1467-9566.2010.01283.x The British Medical Journal (**BMJ**), published the results of a randomized controlled trial indicating that lessons in the Alexander Technique had longterm benefits for back pain patients, and are more effective than prescriptions for either massage or exercise. While Alexander teachers recommend courses of up to 30 lessons, the **BMJ** study suggested that six lessons, when followed by a prescription for exercise, were approximately 72 per cent as effective as 24 lessons and also retained their effectiveness after one year (Little et al. 2008). The Alexander Technique is a form of bodywork which seeks to educate its pupils to use their bodies more efficiently in everyday movement. It is usually taught in one-to-one sessions between a teacher and pupil, which last between half an hour and 45 minutes. These sessions include activities to make pupils aware that they suffer from what the Technique calls 'faulty sensory awareness' and to enable them to differentiate aspects of their movement and thereby develop more precise awareness of their bodily use. Lessons often include activities such as standing and sitting from a chair, and are generally concluded with 'table work' where, in common with bodywork practices such as massage, pupils lie on the table and their bodies are passively manipulated by the teacher. Somatic techniques such as the Alexander Technique, effect improvement by bringing unconscious habit to conscious critical reflection so that it can be worked on. How the Alexander Technique works is as an embodied practice. The Technique is transmitted through the hands of the Alexander teacher, whose manual adjustments of the pupil convey the sense of the work and how the body / self is to be aligned. Conscious control is an important part of this: the pupil is asked to inhibit, or to 'not react' to a particular stimulus. One of the most common stimuli provided in lessons is a chair, and pupils are asked to practice standing and sitting without collapsing the proper alignment of the head-neck-back relationship, sometimes referred to as the 'central core'. When asked to stand up from a chair, most people shorten their necks and look up, throwing their backs into poor alignment. With the Alexander Technique, the head and neck are directed to go 'forward and up', and they lead the action of the body. "Re-education is not a process of adding something, but of restoring something. It was to meet the need of restoring actual conditions of use and functioning which had been previously experienced and afterwards lost that my technique for the re-education of the use of the self was evolved." -Alexander

Iris W. Hung, Aparna A. Labroo, *From Firm Muscles to Firm Willpower: Understanding the Role of Embodied Cognition in Self-Regulation* **Journal of Consumer Research** 2011 37:1046. The mind and the body are so closely tied together, merely clenching muscles can also activate willpower. Thus simply engaging in these bodily actions, which often result from an exertion of willpower, can serve as a non-conscious source to recruit willpower, facilitate self-control, and improve consumer wellbeing.

SCIENCE v GOD

Barbara Bradley Hagerty, **Fingerprints of God: The Search for the Science of Spirituality** 2009 Penguin. Is spiritual experience real or a delusion? Are there realities that we can experience but not easily measure? Does your consciousness depend entirely on your brain, or does it extend beyond? In **Fingerprints of God**, award-winning journalist Barbara Bradley Hagerty delves into the discoveries science is making about how faith and spirituality affect us physically and emotionally as it attempts to understand whether the ineffable place beyond this world can be rationally — even scientifically — explained. Hagerty interviews some of the world's top scientists to describe what their groundbreaking research reveals about our human spiritual experience. From analyses of the brain functions of Buddhist monks and Carmelite nuns, to the possibilities of healing the sick through directed prayer, to what near-death experiences illuminate about the afterlife, Hagerty reaches beyond what we think we know to understand what happens to us when we believe in a higher power. See also: *Is This Your Brain On God?* (May19 2009)
http://www.npr.org/templates/story/story.php?storyId=110997741

J. Anderson Thomson, Clare Aukofer, **Why We Believe in God(s): A Concise Guide to the Science of Faith** 2011 Pitchstone Publishing. God didn't make man; man made gods. In this volume, J. Anderson Thomson, Jr., MD, with Clare Aukofer, offers a succinct yet comprehensive study of how and why the human mind generates religious belief. Dr. Thomson, a highly respected practicing psychiatrist with credentials in forensic psychiatry and evolutionary psychology, methodically investigates the components and causes of religious belief in the same way any scientist

Laura Kragie, MD: Be the Rainbow • Bridge Heaven and Earth

would investigate the movement of astronomical bodies or the evolution of life over time-that is, as a purely natural phenomenon. Providing compelling evidence from psychology, the cognitive neurosciences, and related fields, he, with Ms. Aukofer, presents an easily accessible and exceptionally convincing case that god(s) were created by man — not vice versa. With this slim volume, Dr. Thomson establishes himself as a must-read thinker and leading voice on the primacy of reason and science over superstition and religion. In Why We Believe in God(s), psychiatrist J. Anderson Thomson Jr. examines the hard-wired psychological factors that make humans predisposed to supernatural belief. There is a growing body of experimental evidence that shows that children are hard wired to have an attachment system to adult caretakers, to perceive mind/body dualism, to sense agency in natural events, etc. All of which lend themselves to belief in a superhuman caretaker, separate from physical reality, who makes things happen for a reason. Science continues to explain things that were once the sole domain of religious belief. Thanks to Thomson, the god of the gaps just became a bit smaller. See also: J. Anderson Thomson, *Why We Believe in God(s): the Science of Faith*
http://www.youtube.com/watch?v=1iMmvu9eMrg

David Van Biema, *What Your Brain Looks Like on Faith* **TIME** Dec14 2007 http://www.time.com/time/health/article/0,8599,1694723,00.html#ixzz1qB1S8gHz Harris and two co-authors ran 360 statements by 14 adult subjects whose brain activities were then scanned by functional magnetic resonance imaging (fMRI) devices. It suggests that within the brain scan, at least, the distinction between objective and subjective is not so clear-cut. Although more complex assertions may get analyzed in so-called "higher" areas of the brain, all seem to get their final stamp of "belief" or disbelief in "primitive" locales traditionally associated with emotions or taste and odor. Even "2 + 2 = 4," on some level, is a question of taste. Thus, the statement "that just doesn't smell right to me" may be more literal than we thought. Harris tested how the brain responded to assertions in seven categories: mathematical, geographic, semantic, factual, autobiographical, ethical and religious. All seven provided some useful data, but only the ones relating to math and ethics produced results clear enough to give a vivid picture of the way the simple and the complex, the subjective and the objective intertwine. Regardless of their content, statements that the subjects believed lit up the ventral medial prefrontal cortex (VMPC), a location in the brain best known for processing reward, emotion and taste. Equally "primitive" areas associated with taste, pain perception and disgust determined disbelief. "False propositions may actually disgust us," Harris writes.

Marc Galanter, *Spirituality, Evidence-Based Medicine, and Alcoholics Anonymous* **Am J Psychiatry** 165:12, December 2008 Spirituality is defined by those deeply felt beliefs that give meaning to a person's life. Although spirituality can be embodied in a religious orientation, it can also be understood as commitment to broader ideals or to the welfare of others. While this concept is familiar to many psychiatrists and to our patients, it is generally not understood on the basis of empirical research. Recent psychological and biomedical findings, however, shed light on the mechanisms that underlie its relevance to clinical psychiatry. Furthermore, related research can be useful in understanding the role spirituality plays in the scientifically grounded clinician's work. For example, Alcoholics Anonymous (AA), a self-designated "spiritual fellowship," is a useful adjunct to the practice of evidence-based addiction medicine. Evidence is developing for a specific role of spirituality in its effectiveness.

Kevin Nelson, **The Spiritual Doorway in the Brain: A Neurologist's Search for the God Experience** 2010 Penguin. The world's leading neurologist on out-of-body and near-death experiences shows that spirituality is as much a part of our basic biological makeup as our sex drive or survival instinct. Nelson has discovered that spiritual experiences take place in one of the most primitive areas of the brain. In this eloquent, inspired, and reverent book, he relates the moving stories of patients and research subjects, brain scan analysis, evolutionary biology, and beautiful examples of transcendence from literature to reveal the machinery in our heads that enables us to perceive miracles — whether you are an atheist, Buddhist, or the most devout Catholic.

Andrew Newberg, Mark Robert Waldman, **How God Changes Your Brain: Breakthrough Findings from a Leading Neuroscientist** 2009 Ballantine. Neuroscientist Andrew Newberg, therapist Mark Robert Waldman, and their research team have concluded that active and positive spiritual belief changes the human brain for the better. What's more, actual faith isn't always necessary: atheists who meditate on positive imagery can obtain similar neurological benefits. **How God Changes Your Brain** offers the following breakthrough discoveries: Not only do prayer and spiritual practice reduce stress and anxiety, but just twelve minutes of meditation per day may slow down the aging process. Contemplating a loving God rather than a punitive God reduces anxiety, depression, and stress and increases feelings of security, compassion, and love. Fundamentalism, in and of itself, is benign and can be personally beneficial, but the anger and prejudice generated by extreme beliefs can permanently damage your brain. Intense prayer and meditation permanently change numerous structures and functions in the brain — altering your values and the way you perceive reality.

Steve Volk, **Fringe-ology: How I Tried to Explain Away the Unexplainable-and Couldn't** 2011 HarperOne. Volk decided to focus his gimlet-eyed tenacity on a new beat: the world of psychics, UFOs, and things that go bump in the night. It's a rollicking ride as Volk introduces us to all sorts of fringe-dwellers, many of them reluctant to admit to their paranormal experiences: a NASA astronaut-turned-mystic, a world-famous psychologist who taught us about dying and then decided death may not exist at all, and brave scientists attempting to verify what mystics have been reporting for millennia. Volk investigates what happens in the brains of people undergoing religious experiences, learns how to control his own dreams, and goes hunting for specters in his family's old haunted house. From his journey into the bizarre, Volk returns with a compelling argument that we need to allow for a middle space, a place where paranormal phenomena can be weird and compelling; raise crucial questions; and, quite possibly, remain unexplainable. He rejects the polarized options the twenty-first century seems to offer us: to passionately embrace or hotly reject, to revere only science or only spirituality. And he underscores, again and again, that by raising our most existential questions — why are we here, are we alone in the universe, and what happens when we die? — paranormal stories are in fact a crucial point of connection. It turns out that these "fringe" experiences strike at the core of what it means to be human.

Theresa Vargas, *An Out-of-Body Experience Could Just Be a Beat Away in Virginia*, February 24 2012
http://www.washingtonpost.com/lifestyle/magazine/at-the-monroe-institute-a-spiritual-experience-could-just-be-a-beat-

Laura Kragie, MD: Be the Rainbow • Bridge Heaven and Earth

away/2012/01/27/gIQA9RdrXR_story.html?hpid=z6

Richard Dawkins, **Unweaving the Rainbow: Science, Delusion and the Appetite for Wonder** 2000 Mariner Books. Why do poets and artists so often disparage science in their work? For that matter, why does so much scientific literature compare poorly with, say, the phone book? After struggling with questions like these for years, biologist Richard Dawkins has taken a wide-ranging view of the subjects of meaning and beauty in **Unweaving the Rainbow**, a deeply humanistic examination of science, mysticism, and human nature. Notably strong-willed in a profession of bet-hedgers and wait-and-seers, Dawkins carries the reader along on a romp through the natural and cultural worlds, determined that "science, at its best, should leave room for poetry." -*Amazon Review* "Keats complained that Newton's experiments with prisms had destroyed all the poetry of the rainbow. Not so, says Oxford biologist Dawkins (The Selfish Gene) who, in an eloquent if prickly defense of the scientific enterprise, calls on the "two cultures" of science and poetry to learn from each other." - **Publisher's Weekly Review**

John Keats, 37. *Lamia* Part II **The Poetical Works of John Keats** 1884.

… Do not all charms fly

At the mere touch of cold philosophy?

There was an awful rainbow once in heaven:

We know her woof, her texture; she is given

In the dull catalogue of common things.

Philosophy will clip an Angel's wings,

Conquer all mysteries by rule and line,

Empty the haunted air, and gnomed mine

Unweave a rainbow, as it erewhile made

The tender-person'd Lamia melt into a shade.

Laura Kragie, MD: Be the Rainbow • Bridge Heaven and Earth

Robert Pirsig, **Zen and the Art of Motorcycle Maintenance: An Inquiry into Values** 1974 William Morrow. A narration of a summer motorcycle trip undertaken by a father and his son, **Zen and the Art of Motorcycle Maintenance** becomes a personal and philosophical odyssey into fundamental questions on how to live. The book describes a 17-day journey on his motorcycle from Minnesota to California by the author and his son Chris, joined for the first nine days by close friends John and Sylvia Sutherland. The trip is punctuated by numerous philosophical discussions, referred to as Chautauquas by the author, on topics including epistemology, ethical emotivism and the philosophy of science. Many of these discussions are tied together by the story of the narrator's own past self, who is referred to in the third person as Phaedrus (after Plato's dialogue). Phaedrus, a teacher of creative and technical writing at a small college, became engrossed in the question of what defines good writing, and what in general defines good, or "quality". His philosophical investigations eventually drove him insane, and he was subjected to electroshock treatment, which permanently changed his personality. Pirsig shows that rationality's pursuit of "Pure Truths" derives from the first Greek philosophers who were establishing the concept of truth, against the opposing force of "The Good". He argues that although rational thought may find truth (or The Truth) it may not be valid for all experiences. Therefore, what is needed is an approach to viewing life that is more varied and inclusive and has a wider range of application. He makes a thorough case that originally the Greeks did not distinguish between "Quality" and "Truth" – they were one and the same – and that the divorce was, in fact, artificial (though needed at the time) and is now a source of much frustration and unhappiness in the world, particularly overall dissatisfaction with modern life. Pirsig aims towards a perception of the world that embraces both sides, the rational and the romantic. This means encompassing "irrational" sources of wisdom and understanding as well as science, reason and technology. In particular, this must include bursts of creativity and intuition that seemingly come from nowhere and are not rationally explicable. Pirsig seeks to demonstrate that rationality and Zen-like "being in the moment" can harmoniously coexist. He suggests such a combination of rationality and romanticism can potentially bring a higher quality of life.

Laura Kragie, MD: Be the Rainbow • Bridge Heaven and Earth

Mata Amatanandamayi Devi: primarily known simply as Amma ("Mother"), is a Hindu spiritual leader and guru, who is revered as a saint by her followers. She is widely respected for her humanitarian activities. She is sometimes referred to as "The Hugging Saint". http://en.wikipedia.org/wiki/Mata_Amritanandamayi

TENSEGRITY

R. Buckminster Fuller, **SYNERGETICS — Explorations in the Geometry of Thinking**, Volumes I & II, 1975, 1979 Macmillan Publishing Co. What is tensegrity? "The word 'tensegrity' is an invention: a contraction of 'tensional integrity.' Tensegrity describes a structural-relationship principle in which structural shape is guaranteed by the finitely closed, comprehensively continuous, tensional behaviors of the system and not by the discontinuous and exclusively local compressional member behaviors. Tensegrity provides the ability to yield increasingly without ultimately breaking or coming asunder" - Richard Buckminster Fuller

Timothy Wilken, *Push & Pull* http://www.synearth.net/TensegrityHtml/Tensegrity.html Tensegrity is the pattern that results when push and pull have a win-win relationship with each other. The pull is continuous and the push is discontinuous. The continuous pull is balanced by the discontinuous push producing an integrity of tension — compression. Fuller explained that these fundamental phenomena were not opposites, but compliments that could always be found together. He further explained that push is divergent while the pull is convergent.

Tensegrity structures are structures based on the combination of a few simple but subtle and deep design patterns. Because of these patterns, no structural member experiences a bending moment. This can produce exceptionally rigid structures for their mass and for the cross section of the components. http://en.wikipedia.org/wiki/Tensegrity

The Tensegrity of Carlos Castaneda: Tensegrity is also term used by Carlos Castaneda to refer to some movements called 'magical passes' (a series of meditative stretches, stances and movements) that he said were developed by Native American shamans who lived in Mexico in times prior to the Spanish conquest. Castaneda said that he borrowed the term tensegrity from architecture because the magical passes combine tension and relaxation of the muscles, joints and ligaments in a way that yields a stronger, more flexible, and more "aware" physical body. In conjunction with the gross movements, this is accomplished through a series of proposed metaphysical relationships. Castaneda lays claim that the ancient sorcerers of Mexico conceived of two bodies comprising the human being — one physical, and one made of energy. The consolidation of these bodies is thought to increase vitality and awareness. Further, these two bodies are connected by what he calls the "assemblage point". This point is located about one hand's distance behind the shoulder blades. It is said to be the place where our perception originates, and thus, it determines the ways in which one perceives oneself. Through the practice of Tensegrity, one learns how to displace the assemblage point in different locations and how to change one's perception. This shift of perception involves assuming personal responsibility for one's affairs and allows for a more complete view of interactions. Tensegrity also refers to the adaptation of our own energy to the energy of our surroundings and our fellow beings. http://en.wikipedia.org/wiki/Tensegrity_(Castaneda)

MYTHOLOGY and the RAINBOW

Rainbows are phenomena of light, its perception by the physical senses and the conceptual mind which produces the appearance of a spectral band of colors, often apparently high in the sky, but also at times in close proximity to the observer. The spectrum of colors produced is also itself referred to as the rainbow, and is associated with similar optical phenomena, such as halos, glories, and iridescence. It is widely used symbolically in ways denoting harmonious unity of purpose amidst diversity by various ethnic, religious and other social groups, and as a sign of a divine covenant, being, or bridge between mortal and immortal realms in various cultures. http://en.wikiquote.org/wiki/Rainbows

Lorena Laura Stookey, **Thematic Guide To World Mythology** 2004 ABC-CLIO. For Buddhists, the rainbow is, "the highest state achievable before attaining Nirvana, where individual desire and consciousness are extinguished."

Raymond L. Lee, Alistair B. Fraser, **The Rainbow Bridge: Rainbows in Art, Myth, and Science** 2001 Pennsylvania State Univ Press. Throughout history the rainbow has been seen primarily as a symbol — of peace, covenant, or divine sanction — rather than as a natural phenomenon. Lee and Fraser discuss the role the rainbow has played in societies throughout the ages, contrasting its guises as a sign of optimism, bearer of Greek gods' messages of war and retribution, and a symbol of the Judeo-Christian bridge to the divine. The authors traverse the bridges between the rainbow's various roles as they explore its scientific, artistic, and folkloric visions. God establishes his covenant with Noah and his sons and with all living things, and places the rainbow in the clouds, "the sign of the covenant that I have established between me and all flesh that is on the earth." (Genesis 9-13). In Norse mythology, Bifröst or Bilröst is a burning rainbow bridge that reaches between Midgard (the world) and Asgard, the realm of the gods. In Greek mythology, Iris is the personification of the rainbow and messenger of the gods. As the sun unites Earth and Heaven, Iris links the gods to humanity. She travels with the speed of wind from one end of the world to the other, and into the depths of the sea and the underworld.

Edmund Burke, **A Philosophical Inquiry into our Ideas of the Sublime** 2008 (reissue) Oxford Univ Press. An eloquent and sometimes even erotic book, the Philosophical Enquiry was long dismissed as a piece of mere juvenilia. However, Burke's analysis of the relationship between emotion, beauty, and art form is now recognized as not only an important and influential work of aesthetic theory, but also one of the first major works in European literature on the Sublime, a subject that has fascinated thinkers from Kant and Coleridge to the philosophers and critics of today.

RAINBOW MAN PETROGLYPHS

Indalgo Rainbow Man: The Indalo is a prehistoric symbol found in the "Cave of the Signboard" (La Cueva de Los Letreros) located in the northern province of Almeria, Spain. The Indalo pictograph shows a human with arms stretched above his head holding the arc of a rainbow. In the present village of Mojácar, people paint the symbol with red ocher on houses and over doorways to protect them from storms, lightening and the 'evil eye', Los Taumaturgos (miracle-workers), tell people the symbol has a good energy field surrounding the symbol and it will extend life.

Zuni Rainbow Warrior: Zuni Indians Rainbow Man was found on a Zuni war shield, a symbol of protection. Noted are the outstretched arms, stance of the legs, and the "Bow of Sky Rainbow" above.

Ancient Hawaiian Petroglyphs: The Hawaiian petroglyphs are one very old source for the Rainbow Man icon. Other indigenous civilizations, such as Hawaiian Islanders and American Indians, assigned similar meanings to the same type of symbols as the Indalgo drawing. Rock carvings found throughout the Hawaiian Islands show the "Anuenue Wahine" (Rainbow Woman). The open torso suggests the womb and birth canal. She is the wise woman or the woman who sees all. The "Anuenue Kane" (Rainbow Man) has a closed waistline denoting a male figure. "Rainbow Man" depicts a rainbow resting on his shoulders; it represents each person's responsibility to 'shoulder' the task of protecting Mother Earth

LEGISLATED REGULATIONS OF MEDICAL PRACTICES

The 1986 Emergency Medical Treatment and Active Labor Act (EMTALA): The US Congress passed this Act under President Reagan as part of the Consolidated Omnibus Budget Reconciliation Act. It requires hospitals to provide care to anyone needing emergency healthcare treatment regardless of citizenship, legal status or ability to pay. There are no reimbursement provisions. Participating hospitals may only transfer or discharge patients needing emergency treatment under their own informed consent, after stabilization, or when their condition requires transfer to a hospital better equipped to administer the treatment.
http://en.wikipedia.org/wiki/Emergency_Medical_Treatment_and_Active_Labor_Act

The Patient Protection and Affordable Care Act (PPACA): informally referred to as Obamacare, is a United States federal statute signed into law by President Barack Obama on March 23, 2010. The law (along with the Health Care and Education Reconciliation Act of 2010) is the principal health care reform legislation of the 111th United States Congress. PPACA requires individuals not covered by employer- or government-sponsored insurance plans to maintain minimal essential health insurance coverage or pay a penalty unless exempted for religious beliefs or financial hardship, a provision commonly referred to as the "individual mandate". The Act also

reforms certain aspects of the private health insurance industry and public health insurance programs, increases insurance coverage of pre-existing conditions, expands access to insurance to 30 million Americans, and increases projected national medical spending while lowering projected Medicare spending.
http://en.wikipedia.org/wiki/Patient_Protection_and_Affordable_Care_Act

Accountable care organization (ACO): is a type of payment and delivery reform model that seeks to tie provider reimbursements to quality metrics and reductions in the total cost of care for an assigned population of patients. A group of coordinated health care providers form an ACO, which then provides care to a group of patients. The ACO may use a range of payment models (capitation, fee-for-service with asymmetric or symmetric shared savings, etc.). The ACO is accountable to the patients and the third-party payer for the quality, appropriateness, and efficiency of the health care provided. According to the Centers for Medicare and Medicaid Services, an ACO is "an organization of health care providers that agrees to be accountable for the quality, cost, and overall care of Medicare beneficiaries who are enrolled in the traditional fee-for-service program who are assigned to it."
http://en.wikipedia.org/wiki/Accountable_care_organization

The Health Insurance Portability and Accountability Act of 1996 (HIPAA): Pubic Law 104-191, 110 Stat. 1936, enacted August 21, 1996 by the United States Congress and under President Bill Clinton. Title I of HIPAA protects health insurance coverage for workers and their families when they change or lose their jobs. Title II of HIPAA, known as the Administrative Simplification provisions, requires the establishment of national standards for electronic health care transactions and national identifiers for providers, health insurance plans, and employers. The Administration Simplification provisions also address the security and privacy of health data. The standards are meant to improve the efficiency and effectiveness of the nation's health care system by encouraging the widespread use of electronic data interchange in the U.S. health care system.
http://en.wikipedia.org/wiki/HIPAA

US Food, Drug, and Cosmetic Act (abbreviated as FFDCA, FDCA, or

Laura Kragie, MD: Be the Rainbow • Bridge Heaven and Earth

FD&C): is a set of laws passed by Congress in 1938 giving authority to the U.S. Food and Drug Administration (FDA) to oversee the safety of food, drugs, and cosmetics. In 1968, the Electronic Product Radiation Control provisions were added to the FD&C. Also in that year the FDA formed the Drug Efficacy Study Implementation (DESI) to incorporate into FD&C regulations the recommendations from a National Academy of Sciences investigation of effectiveness of previously marketed drugs. The act has been amended many times, most recently to add requirements about bioterrorism preparations.
http://en.wikipedia.org/wiki/Federal_Food,_Drug,_and_Cosmetic_Act

YEP. THERE'S AN APP FOR THAT"

Some Heaven Helper Apps can be found at the iTunes Store.
http://www.apple.com/itunes/

Here are a few you may want to sample:

Koi Pond

Get High Now

Shakuhachi Meditation Music for Zen Contemplation

Simply Being - Guided Meditation

Rest and Relax - Guided Meditation

Asian Sleep Premium - binaural beats, music, slideshow to enhance sleep

Yogic Breath

Yoga Face

Create Inner Peace: Self Hypnosis

Relax Nature

iYoga

Laura Kragie, MD: Be the Rainbow • Bridge Heaven and Earth

24/7 Chi

Emotional Healing - Lesson and Guided Mediation

Health through Breath: Pranayama

Mindful Moon: Affirmations

iPray: Prayer Times and Qibla Compass

Pocket Prayer Pro: Prayer Journal for Christian

Prayer 2000+ Catholic Prayers by DivineOffice.org

7 Best iPhone and Android Apps for Losing Weight
http://www.thedailybeast.com/galleries/2011/12/24/7-best-iphone-and-android-apps-for-losing-weight.html

ACKNOWLEDGMENTS

This book would not be possible without the generous and insightful feedback from my critical readers. Thank you all, my wonderful posse of beta readers

www.ingramcontent.com/pod-product-compliance
Lightning Source LLC
Chambersburg PA
CBHW051721170526
45167CB00002B/748